SEX SCIENCE SELF

SEX SCIENCE SELF

A Social History
of Estrogen,
Testosterone,
and Identity

BOB OSTERTAG

University of Massachusetts Press

Amherst & Boston

Copyright © 2016 by University of Massachusetts Press
All rights reserved
Printed in the United States of America

ISBN 978-1-62534-213-3 (paper); 212-6 (hardcover)

Designed by Jack Harrison
Set in Adobe Garamond Pro with Huxley Vertical display
Cover design by Kristina Kachele
Cover photograph from Shutterstock © David Smart.

Library of Congress Cataloging-in-Publication Data
Names: Ostertag, Bob, 1957– , author.
Title: Sex science self : a social history of estrogen, testosterone, and identity /
Bob Ostertag.
Description: Amherst : University of Massachusetts Press, [2016] |
Includes bibliographical references and index.
Identifiers: LCCN 2016004219 | ISBN 9781625342133 (pbk. : alk. paper) |
ISBN 9781625342126 (hardcover : alk. paper)
Subjects: | MESH: Gonadal Steroid Hormones | Drug Therapy—history |
Drug Therapy—economics | Sexuality | Transgender Persons | Gender Identity
Classification: LCC QP251 | NLM WK 900 | DDC 612.6—dc23
LC record available at http://lccn.loc.gov/2016004219

British Library Cataloguing-in-Publication Data
A catalogue record for this book is available from the British Library.

to my people,
the freaks and the queers

Contents

Acknowledgments

The list of people who have generously helped me in one way or another with this book is long, and includes queers of all kinds, scholars, doctors, psychiatrists, psychologists, and friends. My deepest thanks to all of you. There are three people who simply must be thanked by name. The first is my editor, Brian Halley, who stuck with this project through thick and thin and was extremely generous with his comments and criticisms, all of which have made the book better than it would have been. The second is my copy editor, Mary Bellino, whose work went far beyond what is usually considered copyediting. The third is my longtime friend Christian Huygen, the founder and director of the Rainbow Heights Club in Brooklyn, New York, the nation's only drop-in social center for LGBT people with severe mental illness diagnoses. Christian has spent I don't know how many hours helping me think through the tangled knot of issues addressed in this book, educating me when needed, pointing me toward other people and resources, shooting down ideas without merit, and patiently answering the phone when I would call at odd hours with some new thought to run by him. That said, I should stress that his generosity does not imply that he agrees with everything in this book. If you ever find yourself in Brooklyn on a late Wednesday afternoon with a little free time and are up for a beautifully queer experience, Wednesday afternoon karaoke at the Rainbow Heights Club is sure to brighten your day.

Words

The boundaries of sexual identities have become increasingly contentious. In this book, I use the words below as defined here:

Transgender refers to people who have taken hormones as a means of "transitioning" from one gender to another, possibly along with "top surgery" for female-to-males, and to all who claim that identity for themselves.

Transexual refers to those who have had "genital sex reassignment" surgery in addition to hormone therapy, and to all who claim that identity for themselves.

Trans is used as an umbrella term for both transgender and transexual.

Gay is used for all those who claim that identity for themselves.

Lesbian is used for all those who claim that identity for themselves.

Queer is used as an umbrella term for all of the above, as well as all others who claim that identity for themselves.

Homosexual is used for men who have sex with men, and women who have sex with women. The term is used mostly when discussing scientific or medical research that employs it.

Bisexual is used for men and women who have sex with both men and women. The term is used mostly when discussing scientific or medical research that employs it.

I make no claim that these usages are the right ones, only that if the subject matter of this book is to be discussed at all then these words must be used, and how they are used should be clearly explained and consistent throughout the text.

SEX SCIENCE SELF

Introduction

My hope is that this book will be useful for anyone who has taken estrogen or testosterone, or considered doing so, for any reason. Given the
sales figures for these products, and the advertising that has accompanied those sales, this includes many millions of Americans.

When I began this project, my interest was more narrowly focused. I
wanted to write a book, first and foremost, for young people wondering
if they should begin hormone treatment in order to undergo what has
become known as "transitioning" between genders. And their families.
And their friends. This group has recently grown far larger than it was
in even the recent past.

This turn to pharmaceuticals is coloring queer culture more generally. Beginning in the 1960s, one of the principle rights demanded by
queer activists was the right to be left alone by doctors. Today, one of
the principle rights demanded by queer activists is the right to receive
medical treatment. This fact alone merits our attention. What were the
causes and what will be the consequences of this about-face? The medical industry is a powerful and complicated beast, with billions of dollars,
entrenched hierarchies of power and authority, and a rapidly expanding
arsenal of technologies. In seeking not to isolate ourselves from that
beast but rather to embrace it more fully, queer culture is changing in
ways both subtle and profound.

But there's more. Estrogen and testosterone, the so-called sex hormones, have become important to the queer community for reasons that
go far beyond their use in transgender "transitioning." The idea that

queers are "born that way" because of prenatal exposure to "sex hormones" has become the foundation on which many of the social and political claims of the community rest—enshrined in judicial rulings, legislation, health insurance policies, and medical practice, emblazoned on t-shirts, banners, and placards, and sung in pop songs. Few are aware that the science behind this claim, currently known as "brain organization theory," is shaky to nonexistent. Even fewer are aware that this same research is routinely invoked for social and political ends many would find appalling. When Lawrence Summers, one of the most powerful men in the nation and at the time the president of Harvard University, provoked a furor by arguing that men outperform women in math and science because of genetic differences between men and women, he was invoking exactly the same research used by queers to claim that they too are "born that way."[1]

As I continued my research, however, I realized that these issues were hardly limited to the queer community. "Sex hormones" have moved to the center of the stories we tell ourselves about not just what makes us transgender, or what makes us homosexual or heterosexual, but what makes us men or women, male or female. Corporate advertising campaigns claim that aging women and men whose bodies produce less "sex hormones" than when they were younger are no longer complete women or men, and sales figures suggest many people believe them. Just one estrogen product generated $1.1 billion in sales in 2013, a year in which the maker jacked up the price 257 percent.[2] Total testosterone sales in 2013 totaled $2.1 billion, and that figure is projected to jump to $3.8 billion a year by 2018, a 158 percent increase in five years.[3]

Taking hormones to amplify, attenuate, or alter your perceived masculinity or femininity has become as American as apple pie. Pro athletes who "dope," gay gym bunnies, US Marines fighting wars in far-off deserts, security guards, cops, bouncers, female politicians, male retirees, transmen, the captains of industry and finance, and high school jocks—all are loading up on *T.* And they are looking across the dance floor at beauty queens, drag queens, prom queens, transwomen, housewives, surrogate mothers, egg donors, women going through menopause, and more—all loaded up on *E.* A businessman in New York City reports that for many young MBAs he knows, "doing T" has become a routine part of getting started in business, as the pace of the work leaves little time for the gym but having a muscular physique can give you that extra edge when you walk into a boardroom. A nationally known husband-and-wife team of yoga teachers take daily "sex hormones" to make them look even more dazzling to their students.[4] *E* and *T* are among the most profitable pharmaceutical products ever sold. So the story told in these pages should be of interest to pretty much anyone engaged with American culture. And since mental health professionals from all over the world come to train in the United States more than to any other country—and carry home with them American notions of gender and sexuality—American beliefs about chemistry and gender are increasingly become the world's beliefs.[5]

Given that pharmaceutical "sex hormones" have become such an important part of life for so many, there has been amazingly little discussion about them. As more and more people in my own social circles began taking them to "transition" their gender, I realized how little I knew about them. But when I asked my friends who were taking them to educate me, they seemed not to know much more than I did. So I began educating myself, and I found that even the doctors who prescribed the stuff knew very little about these substances other than recommended dosages, known side effects, and the like.

This troubled me. Yes, of course, we should know what dose to take, but surely there were bigger questions to ask. The idea that gender has a chemical essence, or that taking a pill can cause one's gender to "transition," are extraordinary claims. They cannot have just fallen from the sky. They must have a long history. Does anyone know it? Doesn't anyone want to learn about it? And what do we really know about the effects of long-term use? Are these well understood?

To my surprise, few even seemed curious about such questions. To the contrary, I encountered more than a little hostility for even asking them. This was especially striking since so much of the intellectual energy fueling transgender activism comes from that part of academia that takes pride in deconstructing ideas scientists take as given. Why were hormones getting a free pass? Beginning from there, I formulated the questions at the heart of this book:

What exactly are estrogen and testosterone? Were these substances discovered or invented? Where did the idea that they are the chemical essence of gender come from? For what other purposes have they been used? Who owns them? Who profits from their sale? What do they actually do in your body? What are the risks of long-term use?

I found that there has indeed been excellent scholarship on the history of "sex hormones." In *Beyond the Natural Body* (1994), Nelly Oudshoorn told of how scientists clung to the belief that there were two "sex hormones," one male and one female, in spite of accumulating evidence that the endocrine system was far more complex than that. Six years later, Anne Fausto-Sterling wrote about the interplay between the development of endocrinology and cultural beliefs about gender and sexuality in *Sexing the Body* (2000). Barbara Seaman, of the Women's Health Action Network, told the story of second-wave feminist activism and estrogen in *The Greatest Experiment Ever Performed on Women* (2003). Seaman's work was followed by Elizabeth Siegel Watkins's *The Estrogen Elixir* (2007). John Hoberman wrote the first scholarly work on the social history of testosterone, *Testosterone Dreams* (2005). Chandak Sengoopta wrote a general "sex hormone" history, *The Most Secret Quintessence of Life* (2006). And these are just the major books.[6]

I was astonished to discover that the words *transgender* and *transsexual* (spelled either with one "s" or two) *do not appear even once in any of these books.* Perhaps this is not surprising. Oudshoorn published her book before *transgender* became a widely used word (yes, widespread use of the term is that recent). Fausto-Sterling, Seaman, and Siegel Watkins are scholars whose primary interest is the complex history of estrogen, women, and feminism, while Hoberman began his research with a focus on athletes and "steroids" (testosterone derivatives). All had good reasons why they might not wish to have their main story get sidetracked in trans issues, which may not have even been on their radar.

But times change, and *transgender* has had a meteoric ascent. The terms *gay* and *lesbian* had been hanging around for many decades before they came to the fore as the publicly embraced identities of a nationally understood subculture in the latter half of the twentieth century. The term *transgender* came into widespread use only in the 1990s, but in just ten years every major Democratic Party presidential candidate officially supported "LGBT rights." During the Barack Obama presidency, LGBT Pride Month was celebrated in the White House every June. What had been the "gay and lesbian press" in the nation's major cities morphed into the "LGBT press," replete with news of the comings and goings of "LGBT people." In 2014, *Time* magazine used its cover to declare that society had reached a "Transgender Tipping Point," illustrated with a stunning photo of the transgender TV star Laverne Cox.[7] In June 2015, *Vanity Fair* published a sensational cover photo from Caitlyn Jenner's first photo shoot as a transwoman. Jenner's tweet "unveiling" the cover broke Internet records when it received a million followers in four hours, eclipsing the opening of even President Obama's Twitter feed weeks before.

The silence of "sex hormone" scholarship on trans history is reciprocated by the silence of trans scholarship on "sex hormone" history. Major books about trans issues began to appear in the mid-1990s, such as Leslie Feinberg's *Transgender Warriors* (1996). The most comprehensive is Joanne Meyerowitz's *How Sex Changed* (2002); Deborah Rudacille's *The Riddle of Gender* (2006) is also excellent. *Transgender History* (2008), by the transgender activist and scholar Susan Stryker, is a historical introduction for a general readership. For primary source material, there is the massive, 752-page *Transgender Studies Reader,* edited by Stryker and Steven Whittle. And we have just scratched the surface.[8]

You could read every page of all these books and never learn that the corporations which own the patents for the major estrogen and testosterone products spent millions of dollars over several decades selling the *idea* that testosterone and estrogen are the chemical essences of masculinity and femininity. You would not learn that contesting this marketing had been a major goal of the feminists of the 1960s and 1970s, and that for many of those women, the first step in resisting the patriarchy was to "take back their bodies" by rejecting the "sex hormone" marketing hype pharmaceutical companies were heaping upon them. Nor would you have any inkling of the decades of research and debate about the safety of long-term use of these products, debates that are anything but settled.

You would learn from transgender histories that Magnus Hirschfeld organized the first documented "sex reassignment" surgeries in Berlin in the early twentieth century, but you would not learn that, at the same time, Hirschfeld was also arranging the first surgeries to "cure" male homosexuals. You would learn all about the long history of reluctance on the part of medical professionals to provide hormones to people who *wanted* to change their sex or gender, but you would learn nothing of the parallel history of medical professionals *forcing* those same hormones on people who did *not* want to change their sex or gender, for the purpose of either "curing" their homosexuality or punishing them for it (or both). When you widen the lens and put the two together, the contrast is stunning. On the one hand, we find a group of people insisting their gender nonconformity was a medical condition that required treatment with hormones which doctors refused to provide for them, and on the other hand, a group of people insisting their gender nonconformity was *not* a medical condition and yet doctors were shoving hormones into their bodies against their will.

You would learn that, in the United States, the doctor who led the crusade for the right to hormone therapy for people who wished to change sex or gender was Harry Benjamin, and you would learn that in 1979 the first professional association for doctors treating transexuals was named the Harry Benjamin International Gender Dysphoria Association in his honor. You would not learn, however, that Benjamin began his career as a self-described "disciple" of Eugen Steinach, an Austrian doctor who became rich and famous claiming that he could rejuvenate aging men by performing vasectomies on them.[9] Or that Benjamin founded the Life Extension Institute in New York City for performing Steinach's bogus rejuvenation surgeries, that he continued to champion those procedures long after everyone else had rejected them, became something of a medical laughingstock as a result, and only switched to trans medical care after his rejuvenation practice collapsed.

You would learn that in 1948, a very unhappy person who would soon become Christine Jorgensen, by far the most famous transperson in history until Caitlyn Jenner, picked up *The Male Hormone,* a blockbuster book by a popular science writer, and found in its pages information that would change her life. "It seemed possible that I was holding salvation in my hands," she later wrote. And within a year, she was ready to begin: "There, at last, the small bottle lay in my hand. How strange it seemed to me that the whole answer might lie in the particular combination of atoms contained in those tiny, aspirin-like pills." But you would not learn of the crucial role *The Male Hormone* played in the early marketing of testosterone as "the most secret quintessence of life" and the wonder drug of masculinity and male rejuvenation.[10]

You would learn that the term *LGBT community* entered US presidential discourse at the end of 2008, but you would not learn that annual sales of testosterone products hit $1 billion at precisely the same time.

And most certainly you would not learn of the long series of medical catastrophes that has resulted from the use of "sex hormones," or the crusading doctors who led their patients off medical cliffs.

The medical fields of endocrinology and gerontology have done their best to forget this troublesome and embarrassing history. As one textbook states, "Just as the editors of Soviet encyclopedias correct historical 'errors' by simply scissoring out entire chapters of previous editions, so gerontology has tried to consign its early deviationists to oblivion."[11] It took scholarship by the likes of Oudshoorn, Fausto-Sterling, Sengoopta, and others to unearth from the field of endocrinology what was buried.

The field of transgender history is so new it is only now being written. Paradoxically, the history of estrogen and testosterone that has recently been excavated from the field of endocrinology is being buried anew in the field of transgender history. Transgender histories too often take "sex hormones" at face value, as the timeless, ahistorical chemical essences of gender. The chemicals simply are what they are, always have been, and always will be. Yet as Oudshoorn observed early on, "Sex hormones are not entities that only had to be 'discovered' in nature . . . [but] were objects constructed in the laboratory as materializations of particular ideas about what sex hormones should look like."[12]

The point is not that we should declare "sex hormones" to be "good" or "bad." The point is that they are at the center of the story, not outside of it. Because the biggest story here—at least in the sense of the story that will have the most consequences for the most people—is not the story of particular kinds of chemicals or people, be they L, G, B or T. It is the story of the nexus between technology and what has come to be called human identity.

The story of the interweaving of human identity and technology is not an easy story to tell, or to hear. It is fraught with highly emotional difficulties that are currently causing enormous stress and anguish in the queer community. Intense emotions surround assertions about who transgender people "really are," and indeed who women and men "really are." For example, there are women who strongly believe that a woman is a specific kind of person, not synonymous with a man who has taken estrogen and perhaps also had genital surgery. They experience such a person's claim to be a woman as a denial of the discrimination, objectification, and even violence they have faced all their lives, and even a negation of their personhood. Likewise, there are those who were born male but who have taken estrogen and perhaps also had surgery, and believe they have become (and in some sense always were) women. They experience rejection of this claim as a denial of the discrimination and even violence they have faced all their lives, and even a negation of their personhood.

Within the transgender community, there is an equally explosive debate as to whether there is a medical pathology at the root of the transgender identity that can be treated with medical technology. Here again, some transgender people hear any assertion that they are somehow "sick" as a denial of the discrimination and violence they have faced all their lives, and even a negation of their personhood, which they feel compelled to resist. Other transgender people hear the assertion that they suffer from no valid medical pathology as a denial of the pain and suffering they have endured, and as discrimination against people with one particular pathology and not another. The bitterness in the confrontation over whether transgender people are "really sick" comes from the fact that the outcome of this debate carries a price tag, in that it heavily influences the question of whether hormones and surgeries for transgender people are covered by health insurance.

The tensions over who transgender people "really are" have recently escalated to the point where some transgender activists and writers have accused women who insist that male-to-female transgender people are not "real women" of engaging in hate speech, and demanded that their organizations be labeled hate groups.[13]

These questions about who transgender people "really are," or who men and women "really are," are not questions that the history I am telling here seeks to answer. Neither is the question of whether transgender people, or for that matter anyone else, are "really sick." I hope that my writing will convey my thoughts accurately enough that this will be clear throughout the text. But given the degree of anger currently swirling around these questions, it is worthwhile to state this explicitly at the outset.

My focus is on the chemical technologies that transgender people use to "transition," and others use to "augment," their gender (men to become more masculine, women to become more feminine). And my question is not what these chemicals "really are" or what they "really mean," but what is their history?

For example, I put the term "sex hormones" in scare quotes. I want to know: Where did the idea that estrogen is female and testosterone male, that chemicals can be masculine or feminine, come from? What research supports it? What research contradicts it? Who proposed it? Who benefits financially from its propagation? My goal is not to finally determine what these chemicals "really are," but to understand the story of how we arrived at the set of beliefs we currently hold about them.

But limiting my focus in this way hardly means this book will not cause controversy. Many people have battled long and hard to win access to these chemicals. Socially and politically, they see access to "sex hormones" as the victory of a gender revolution waged by an oppressed minority that took years of struggle and sacrifice to achieve. Politically, they may perceive any critical examination of them as a negation of their struggle and their victories, and even a denial of the discrimination and violence they experienced that fueled that struggle. Personally, they may believe that this technology caused their gender to "transition." This transition may now be a deep part of who they understand themselves to be, and thus any questioning of the meaning they have assigned to that technology is profoundly threatening.

Even the mere telling of the history of "sex hormones" can be threatening. For the story includes many prior dramatic claims about what these chemicals are and can do. Most of these claims experienced a spectacular rise, and then an equally spectacular fall, often with a belated realization that severe harm was caused to thousands of people. It is difficult to come away from this history with a high degree of confidence that our present-day beliefs and practices surrounding these technologies will prove any more permanent than those that went before. This is at the root of the silence on the history of "sex hormones" in transgender history.

This is why many who read the manuscript of this book expect it to stir up something of a hornet's nest. Sadly, I suspect they may be right. The more prudent reader may then wonder why I nevertheless pursued its publication.

My answer has two parts. Most immediately, as I mentioned earlier, this technology has become so prevalent among my friends and community, yet so little is widely known about it. More broadly, I believe these questions are crucial to our time and place in history. Gender may be the first terrain in which people find their very sense of self leashed to a specific nexus of technology and identity, but it will not be the last.

If that claims sounds overblown, consider that John Hoberman argues that "the 'doping' of athletes with androgens and other hormones" raises philosophical issues that "originate in the most basic questions about what it means to be a human being," and that such technologies "will precipitate an unprecedented crisis of human identity during the twenty-first century."[14] I agree. And while the trail Hoberman followed to this conclusion began in the use of testosterone in sports, there is another trail beginning in the queer community's use of hormones for gender "transitioning" that arrives at the same place.

While the debate about testosterone use in sports centers on what is fair in competition, what are the limits of what counts as human, and—most immediately—the fame and considerable fortunes of the individuals involved, the debate about testosterone use in the queer community has centered on identity and politics. As our ever more powerful technology becomes ever more tightly intertwined with our multiplying identities, people who have engaged with a given technology to construct an identity may perceive any questioning of the meaning they assign to that technology as an assault on their personhood, their very self. As I have noted, they may even feel threatened by the mere telling of the history of previous meanings assigned to these substances, and the associated medical practices that were first hailed as revolutionary before collapsing in tragedy and recrimination.

But we cannot simply declare large swaths of history to be politically out of bounds. I rebel, deeply, at statements that effectively tell us, "Don't study this because it is dangerous to do so." The real danger, I believe, is in ruling some parts of history off limits. Given the current rate of technological change, and the new physical and social terrains that technology is permeating, admonishments to not examine the meanings of technology are particularly dangerous.

We live in the age of global warming, mass extinction, big data, Google Earth, killer drones, smartphones, constant surveillance, and a rapidly growing medicine chest of pharmaceutical products that have become so powerful we now experience them as central to our sense of self. If we are going to find our way in all of this, *all* of it must be open to scrutiny, questioning, and debate. *All* meanings of technology must be on the table, open to examination, and fallible.

I find it profoundly distressing that my community, the queer community, is the first to put forward a political position which asserts that there are certain meanings of technology it is unacceptable to question. That, because of who we are, there are some questions about technology we must not ask.

I came of age in the social and intellectual milieu that the gay liberation movement of the 1960s and 70s left in its wake. One of the ways in which "gay liberation" differed from the queer activism that came after was the belief that the queer experience could make a unique contribution to the broader movement for liberation, equality, and ecology of the time. The activism of the 1950s was narrowly focused on winning basic legal rights for homosexuals, even the right simply to exist. The activists of the 1960s and 1970s saw the bigger liberation movements of the era and wanted to jump on board, to add a queer perspective.

Since then, what has become known as the LGBT community has narrowed its gaze back down to specific legal rights like the right to marry or serve in the US military, and access to pharmaceutical drugs and other medical technologies. The issues discussed in this book, however, open a window onto a much larger landscape. Can we find a way to respect those whose sense of self is deeply intertwined with particular beliefs about particular technologies while at the same time leaving those beliefs and technologies open to question? If we can do this, we will indeed be making a contribution to a society in which many others will be confronting new variations of this same dilemma in the near future. If we cannot, we will be doing no one a favor, least of all ourselves.

One measure for how well we succeed will be how freely we can study and discuss our own history.

I originally intended to leave myself out of this introduction, but several of my younger friends and colleagues who were kind enough to offer their suggestions were adamant in their advice to the contrary. They argued that since there is no neutral place from which to tell a story, and in

consideration of the tensions in this particular story, readers will want to
know in advance who I am and why this is the story I wish to tell. Since
I care deeply that this story be heard, I have followed their advice. But if,
like me, you think people who begin narratives about events of historic
importance by talking about themselves are yet another indicator of the
narcissism of our times, please skip ahead to the beginning of the next
section. You can always come back to this part later.

The dedication with which the book begins, "to my people, the freaks
and the queers," is sincere. My own life—emotional, romantic, artistic,
intellectual, social, and sexual—has been rooted in the queer community, and my loves have been multiply transgressive: interracial, inter-
generational, with lesbians, gays, and bisexuals, drag queens, effeminate
fags, and butch dykes. A butch lesbian lover and I made a baby together
in the 1980s (something not so out of the ordinary now but way out of
bounds back then). My daughter grew up raised by her two moms in one
house and myself and a drag queen in another a block away.

My previous books have covered guerrilla media activism, the history
of social justice movements, art and politics, and labor organizing in Las
Vegas.[15] In all cases I have tried to make my scholarship immediately
and practically useful to the communities in which I live.

I am fifty-nine years old, which means I was twelve (and living in a
sleepy Colorado town) at the time of the Stonewall riot. I missed the gay
liberation years by a generation.

I was twenty-four and living in Manhattan in 1981 when the first
AIDS cases among gay men were reported. I largely missed the earliest years of the epidemic, however, as I was completely absorbed in the
revolutionary movement in El Salvador. It was there that I learned to
write, first as the publisher and editor of the newspaper of the US soli-
darity movement, and then as a journalist covering the war for progres-
sive newspapers around the world. I left the Salvadoran movement at the
end of the eighties, but have remained involved in political projects of
various kinds ever since.

As a young "freak" in the late 1960s and early 1970s, I was touched by
the gender upheaval of the time. In my case, this revolved around long
hair. No, we did not talk about "destabilizing the gender binary," but
long hair on males and pants on females were highly contested assaults
on exactly that, and were understood as such at the time. The only time I

was ever in a fight was in junior high school, when I defended an effeminate male friend who had the longest hair in the school from a bunch of boys who had brought sheep shears to school and tried to pin him down on the playground to forcibly cut his hair, which they understood to be a flagrant transgression of gender norms. One year later I was threatened at knifepoint by a gang of young men who referred to me as a girl because of the length of my hair.

Like all the "freaks" of the era, I perused the pages of the *Whole Earth Catalog*, the operating manual of the counterculture, which ran articles on how to determine the age of a cow and build composting toilets next to ads for the earliest personal computers and music synthesizers. I was enthralled by all of it. The core idea was that "appropriate technology" would make society more democratic and ecologically sustainable. But the people and ideas that launched the *Catalog* spawned personal computers and today's Silicone Valley, just down the road from my home in San Francisco. I used a personal computer to write this book, but I now view my early beliefs about technology as naive. I have learned to place claims about the social benefits of new technologies, even "small" or "appropriate" technology, under far more scrutiny than I used to. Not just because those claims are usually false, but because as technology comes to dominate more and more of our lives, how we handle the choices it creates, and the meanings we ascribe to those choices, become a central part of who we are.

Today, I am as ensnared in the contradictions of life in the pharmaceutical age as anyone. My chemicals of choice today begin with a daily three-pill HIV "cocktail." When I was diagnosed with HIV in 1993, I was told I had just a few more years to live. In all likelihood, without these newly synthesized chemicals produced for profit by giant capitalist enterprises, I would not be alive to write this book. My morning pill regimen also includes yet another newly synthesized chemical sold for a tidy sum by a giant corporation, called an antidepressant. The effects of antidepressants are poorly understood and fiercely debated among specialists. Some believe the drugs' effect on depression to be entirely placebo in character, while others doubt that depression as it is currently understood "even exists." I have extremely ambivalent feelings about these drugs myself and as a result have stopped using them several times, always with very unhappy results. When I see my transgender

friends also taking pills about which there are similarly heated, unresolved debates over whether the drugs do anyone any good, and whether
the disease they are intended to treat "even exists," I am struck by how
much their experiences have in common with my own. Thus, if at any
point in this book the writing seems to suggest that I see myself as above
the pharmaceutical fray, that is my mistake, not my intention.

Identity and Hormones

This book is not a transgender history. But some brief remarks on certain aspects of that history that will be very important to our story are
in order.

The blazing rise of the trans identity has been matched by the in-
tensity of controversies over what the identity actually means and who
it includes. The story begins at the end of the 1960s, when a tireless
activist and small-scale publisher named Virginia Prince "coined the
words *transgenderism* and *transgenderist* as nouns describing people like
myself who have breasts and live full time as a woman, but who have
no intention of having genital surgery." Prince went to great lengths to
distinguish *transgender* from homosexual and transexual. She founded
the world's first transgender organization, which explicitly banned "homosexuals, transsexuals or emotionally disturbed people" from joining.
To make her disdain for homosexuals even more pointed, she titled her
first book *The Transvestite and His Wife*. As for transexuals, she claimed
that "sex reassignment surgery is a communicable disease" that is spread
to gullible transvestites by sensational media reports.[16]

By the end of the 1990s, many of those who had come to embrace
the transgender identity had come to see gays, lesbians, and bisexuals
as allies. Instead of standing defiantly off to the side, the "T" migrated
over and was ultimately appended to "LGB." But within the transgender community itself, agreement on what the word actually meant remained elusive. Fifteen years later, increasingly bitter controversies about
its meaning had come to dominate much of the discussion within the
transgender social world.

In her 2008 book *Transgender History*, the historian Susan Stryker
rigorously reviewed these disparate groupings and claims. This required
spending the first twenty pages simply laying out contradictory and

overlapping terms and definitions, before concluding that "there is no way of using the word [transgender] that doesn't offend some people by including them where they don't want to be included or excluding them from where they want to be included." Stryker decided that the only way to proceed would be to sidestep the problem by using the term to refer to any "practice or identity [that] crosses gender boundaries that are considered socially normative in the contemporary United States."[17]

I will return to Stryker's work in the pages that follow. Much of the "science" on which the political claims of transgender activists—and increasingly the claims of all LGBT activists—are founded is based on the assumption that the presence of transgender people (or homosexuals, bisexuals, lesbians, or gays, or straights) within a sample group can be precisely counted. In evaluating this research, it will serve us well to remember that the most rigorous review by the most prominent transgender historian concluded that such counting is impossible.

I observed these developments in my own social world. When I moved to San Francisco in the 1980s, transgender was a term I heard rarely if at all, even though my social circle centered on the most consciously gender-transgressive part of the queer community. Today many of my peers consider themselves transgender. And when I question them about the precise meaning of the term, I hear the same debate and disagreement Stryker summarizes in her book.

Despite all the confusion and animosity, when I listen closely to those around me, particularly the younger queers in their twenties and thirties, I find there *is* a more specific meaning of transgender that has in fact come into common vernacular in the sexual subcultures of the major urban centers where such things are adjudicated. In actual conversational practice, *transgender* often refers to people who take hormones to modify their bodies: female-bodied people who take testosterone, and male-bodied people who take estrogen. The former may also possibly undergo a double mastectomy ("top surgery"), and the latter may also opt for surgical breast implants, but this is not required. People who go further and engage in genital surgery are generally referred to as *transsexual.*

This meaning of *transgender* was precisely articulated in Justin Vivian Bond's 2011 essay announcing Bond's "embracing of trans identity."[18]

Bond had been an internationally known cabaret star for decades, and an icon of gender transgression and fluidity in the queer underground. Bond identified at times as a gay man, as a drag queen, and most often simply as a *tranny* (a term that gained favor in the 1990s among the gender queer as a term of endearment, but is now increasingly rejected as "transphobic" by a younger generation). In the essay, Bond is explicit about the relation between the transgender identity and hormone therapy: "I am beginning hormone treatments not to become a woman but in order to actualize what I've always known myself to be—a trans person. I want my body to be a declaration and physical manifestation of my transgendered spirit."[19]

Bond is hardly alone. One could make a long list of well-known people who began public life as "gay" or "lesbian" but then switched to "transgender," and in almost every case the change of identity corresponds with the beginning of hormone treatment.[20]

Debates about the source of the transgender identity are just as fierce and unresolved as the debates over who it includes. The dominant position today holds that one's gender identity, one's sense of self as male or female, is determined by the chemical processes in a mother's body while a fetus is still in the womb. At the other extreme, Susan Stryker argues that people become transgender when they choose to engage with technology: "It's about trying to speak from this embodied place that is technologically constructed."[21] Yet as we will see over the course of this book, these are just different ways of talking about hormones. One position focuses on the hormones produced by a mother's body, or entering the mother's body through pharmaceutical drugs or environmental sources.[22] Stryker focuses on hormones produced by giant pharmaceutical corporations and taken deliberately at some time after birth. But as disparate as these positions appear at first blush, all agree that hormones are what make a transperson trans.

When I began to formulate the ideas for this book, I did a series of interviews in which I pursued this notion that hormones are the defining factor. A high-profile trans-identified doctor whose practice includes mostly trans patients told me that his infallible method for distinguishing "real transpeople" from wannabes was to see whether they were willing to take the full dosage of hormones he prescribes. If patients take just half of the daily dose, so that the changes in their bodies occur more gradually, he diagnoses them as not "really" transgender. Here the equation of trans-ness with hormones is not only explicit but *quantifiable:* a "real" transperson takes a certain dose of hormones; those who take a lesser dose are less than trans.[23]

I went directly from that interview to an interview with Sam, a young transman who is centrally involved in trans activism in San Francisco. Sam told me that he himself was one of those who took a half-dose of hormones. He said that he had watched others in his social circle begin testosterone therapy and lose their femininity so fast that the experience was traumatic, so Sam wanted to take his time. He felt insulted that a doctor who was himself transgender would dismiss Sam's trans identity on that basis, and drew immediate connections from the doctor's diagnostic procedure to how hormones and identity are understood by his friends. "*Theoretically* my understanding is that to my generation transgender means the explosion of all boxes," he told me. "But my *experience* in my social circle is that transgender means that you need to have made the rite of passage of doing hormones. It seemed like if I was not going to do hormones then transgender wasn't the term for me."[24]

I later had a conversation with another young transman in New York City about these same issues. When I mentioned that the only thing I could find consistent in how transpeople actually use the term "trans" was to refer to people who take hormones to modify their bodies, he objected, "But I don't know *anybody* who thinks that." Later in the conversation, I told him about Sam's decision to do a half dose of hormones at a time. "Well," he replied, with no sense of irony, "maybe he's not *really trans.*"

The contradiction Sam describes dates back to the early 1990s and the activist group Queer Nation. The militants of Queer Nation deliberately promoted "queer" as a way to bring the multiplying identities of the sexual subculture under a single all-inclusive term focused more on what people had in common than what divided them. Queer Nation was structured as a collection of affinity groups, and in 1992 a transgender affinity group formed in San Francisco's Queer Nation chapter. Queer Nation faded from the scene not long after, but the transgender affinity group continued as Transgender Nation, linking similar affinity groups in other cities. Transgender activism took off, and instead of replacing the acronym LGB with the single word *queer,* the accepted acronym has expanded even further to LGBT, and sometimes LGBTQ—with Q as yet another letter rather than an umbrella to encompass all.

As Sam noted, the term *transgender* has to some degree begun to function in the way that the founders of Queer Nation hoped *queer* would: an identity that, in Sam's words, "explodes all boxes." Or in Susan Stryker's words, includes any "practice or identity [that] crosses gender boundaries that are considered socially normative in the contemporary United States." Yet this "theoretical" definition exists in acute tension with what Sam finds to be the social reality in San Francisco and other queer urban centers: if you are not ready to go through "the rite of passage" of hormone therapy, then transgender is not the term for you.

That chemical rite of passage has thus become a central focus for a new generation of young people who feel themselves to be outside the mainstream of gender expression and sexual attraction. As Sam recounts, "Technology, body modification—there is a total exotification of it. When I went from girl to dyke I got about 125 percent more ass. When I went to trans guy I got another 125 percent. I don't think that is why I did it, but people definitely exotify it." The question of whether or not to take hormones is now part and parcel of the coming out process.

The chemical rite of passage now has its own word, *transition,* as in transition from male to female, or vice versa. The underlying belief is that bodies or people don't have gender, chemicals do. Estrogen is female, testosterone is male. Bodies are understood to be blank slates on which maleness or femaleness can be chemically inscribed.

This book can be considered a history of that idea: where and when it emerged; the political, economic, social, and personal interests that shaped and reshaped it; and how it came to such a place of prominence today.

Since I hope this history will be useful to so many, I have written in conversational English, and I have found it adequate to the task. The book would not be any more nuanced had it been written in the stylized prose of "critical theory." It would only have been more difficult for those outside of that specialty to follow.

The issues at the heart of this book are historical. But within academia, study of queer and transgender issues is often viewed through the lens of critical theory. As a result, what students learn runs heavy on philosophy and light on history. Students at many colleges and universities can major in Queer Theory or Gender Studies and graduate with the ability to wield obscure philosophical vocabulary, while remaining unaware of most or all of the basic history recounted in this book. For example, many more are able to carry on a nuanced conversation about the philosophy of gender identity than are aware that the belief that testosterone is a "male" and estrogen a "female" chemical—beliefs so widely accepted today—are the result of decades of advertisement and promotion by the corporations who profit from the sale of those chemicals. This emphasis on philosophy or "theory" to the detriment of history is not serving our community well, and I hope this book will be at least a nudge in the other direction.

I am not an endocrinologist. I learned almost everything I know about endocrinology while researching this book. In doing so I relied extensively, though not entirely, on secondary sources. In other words, if you look through the citations in this book, while you will find many interviews I did and medical journal articles I read, you will also find many books written by others, in which the writers of those books cite interviews they did and medical journal articles they read. As I noted earlier, I am not so much writing a new history here as creating a synthesis of two fields of historical scholarship that have been kept in mutual isolation.

Complex Systems in the Human Body

Finally, a proviso. Hormones that are biologically produced in our bodies are considered part of the *endocrine system.* This system includes *hormones,* or chemicals that circulate in our blood, the organs that secrete them, and receptors they bind to. The endocrine system was originally thought to involve just a few organs secreting a small number of hormones, including what was hypothesized to be "the male hormone" secreted by the testicles, and "the female hormone" secreted by the ovaries. As with so many natural systems, however, the endocrine system has proven to be far more complex than initially thought. At current count there are about fifty hormones. These are secreted by the pineal gland, pituitary gland, pancreas, ovaries, testes, thyroid gland, parathyroid gland, hypothalamus, gastrointestinal tract, and adrenal glands, and even the kidney, liver, and heart. The pituitary gland regulates all other glands, and it is itself regulated by the brain. So the brain is now considered part of the endocrine system as well. The endocrine system is currently the subject of a considerable amount of research, and the more we learn, the more we become aware of how little we understand about it.

When a hormone binds to a receptor, a physiological process is triggered, and a lot of what happens in our bodies is thus regulated by hormones. The endocrine system involves multiple exceedingly complex *feedback loops,* which serve to keep the amount of hormones circulating in our blood within ranges that stimulate physiological processes in ways we consider healthy.

The endocrine system is not the only system in our bodies that uses feedback loops to stay within a healthy range. All warm-blooded creatures, for example, have a self-regulatory control function that keeps their body temperature within a certain range. Their bodies use a feedback loop: if the temperature swings too high or too low, processes kick in that try to bring it back into line. As everyone knows, human bodies self-regulate to an internal temperature of 98.6°F.

Except not really. There is in fact no single number that represents a "normal" or "healthy" temperature for all people in all circumstances. So where did 98.6 come from? Some surmise that two hundred years ago Gabriel Fahrenheit might have originally used human body temperature as a reference point for the temperature scale that bears his name, defining human body temperature as 100°F, but no one really knows. At any rate, the Fahrenheit scale was later revised to use the boiling point of water as its reference, causing the alleged normal body temperature to drift. In 1861, Carl Reinhold August Wunderlich claimed to have measured the armpit temperatures of 25,000 people, and he reported the mean to be 98.6 °F. But Wunderlich's thermometers were not calibrated to any standard, and he did not indicate how his results were calculated.[25]

The latest (but not final) word on the subject is that "normal" body temperatures differ from individual to individual, as well as by time of day, season, and activity. Nevertheless, 98.6 is the undisputed *cultural* norm, indelibly inscribed in our understanding of our bodies. It is the title of several pop songs, a country western song, a male vocal group, a book on survival and preparedness, two novels, a book on meditation, and so on. Though if we happened to have lived in the former Soviet bloc, the magic number glorified in literature and song would have been 97.9.

The story of human body temperature provides a neat example of a system in the human body that was initially thought to be simple and fully understood but turned out to be complex and is still not fully explained. Yet in popular culture, as well as in medical clinics and even in some research labs, it is considered a settled matter with one right answer. It is just the sort of thing the medical historian Anne Fausto-Sterling had in mind when she noted, "A scientific fact, once established, may sometimes be disproved in one field, remain a 'fact' in others, and have a further life in the popular mind."[26]

I

Before Pharmaceuticals

The idea that testicles are somehow the source of manhood goes back to the far reaches of recorded history. Millennia before the discovery of chemicals, before anyone suspected that blood could be broken down into component compounds which regulate bodily function, it was understood that male castration (the removal or crushing of the testicles) had physiological, behavioral, and social consequences. Eunuchs, or castrated males, can be found in history across thousands of years and many cultures, sometimes in very large numbers scarcely imaginable to present-day sensibilities. Though each culture had its own unique social role for eunuchs, in all cases eunuchs were thought to be something less than a man.

Eunuchs, Testicles, and Ovaries

Thousands upon thousands of males were made eunuchs for political reasons in political systems in which absolute power resided in the body of one man. Since the first obligation of the ruler was to produce a male heir, many such cultures independently concluded that one way to safeguard the ruler from the devious schemes of usurpers was to castrate the men surrounding him. Not only were eunuchs unable to sire children who might aspire to the throne, they were seen as less of a sexual threat with regard to the ruler's wife, or wives, or harem. Eunuchs were also believed to be less ambitious, and were often of such lowly social status that they could be put to death without much fuss should circumstances require. The historical record of eunuchs stretches all the way back into prehistory. Indeed, the creation of eunuchs by castration has been described as "almost certainly the first experiment in endocrinology." Assyrian kings, Egyptian pharaohs, Roman emperors, and Ottoman sultans all surrounded themselves with eunuchs.[1]

There is also a long history of religious eunuchs, including a Christian tradition that runs from the earliest days of the Church right into the twentieth century. According to the New Testament, an Ethiopian eunuch was the first Gentile to convert to Christianity. And there were musical eunuchs, or *castrati* (male vocalists castrated before puberty to keep their singing voice in the soprano range), which in the West are documented from late antiquity until the practice was outlawed in Italy in the 1870s. The testicles of some five thousand European boys were either crushed or removed for musical purposes in every year of the eighteenth century. The most famous *castrati* attained the status of cultural icons—the rock stars of their day—and Italian opera fans would greet their performances with cries of *"Viva il coltello!"* (Long live the knife!).[2]

If removing a man's testicles made him less than a man, it stood to reason that adding more testicles might make him more of a man, and there is an equally long and varied history of using animal testicles to pump up manhood. Greeks and Romans used wolf and goat testes as sexual stimulants.[3] More than a millennium later, in London in 1696, William Salmon's landmark *Dispensatory* recommended a variety of animal testes for both men's and women's complaints: boar testicles to treat "weakeness and barrenness," dog testicles to induce "lust" and "dried deer testicles drunk in wine" for the same purpose, horse testicles to "excite venery and expel the afterbirth," leopard testicles to help a woman "provoke the terms," badger testicles eaten with honey to aid fertility, buzzard testicles to "help the weakness of generation," eagle testicles for venery, and testicles of eagles, buzzards, and sturgeon for similar purposes.[4] Testicular cures fell out of favor in the eighteenth century and then, as we will see, were revived with a vengeance in the late nineteenth and early twentieth centuries.

As for women and womanhood, today's fascination with ovaries is of comparatively recent origin, in part because the location of ovaries in the body makes them more difficult to identify, examine, remove, or even find than testicles. But beliefs about the ways and means of human reproduction were also a barrier to the cultural rise of the ovaries. Aristotle described the practice of excising the ovaries of sows "with the view of quenching in them sexual appetites and of stimulating growth in size and fatness," implying an understanding that the presence or absence of ovaries had both behavioral and physiological consequences.[5] But Aristotle and his contemporaries believed in the "seed and soil" concept of reproduction: the male provided the "seed" and the female the "soil." Whatever that soil was, its connection to ovaries was hardly obvious, and there is no record of removing or adding ovaries in women to parallel the long history of men and their testicles. Ancient medicine located the root of femininity not in the ovaries but in the uterus. It was only with the discovery of the ovum in 1827 that the ovary displaced the uterus as the defining organ of femininity. By 1848 the German physician Rudolf Virchow declared: "The female is female because of her reproductive glands. All her characteristics of body and mind, of nutrition and nervous activity, the sweet delicacy and roundedness of limbs[,] . . . the development of the breasts and non-development of the vocal organ, the beauties of her hair and the soft down on her body, those depths of feeling, that unerring intuition, that gentleness, devotion, and loyalty— in short, all that we respect and admire as truly feminine, are dependent on the ovaries. Take the ovaries away and we get the repulsive, coarsely formed, large-boned, moustached, deep-voiced, flat-breasted, resentful, and egoistic virago (*Mannweib*)."[6]

Animal Spirits, Hydraulics, and Electricity

Though testicles had long been identified as the source of manhood, the understanding of *how* these two little globs of tissue did the trick went through several revisions. Alexandrian physicians in the third century BC proposed that "animal spirits" were responsible: weightless, invisible entities that flowed through the body regulating its functions. The theory was persuasive, and "animal spirits," or "humors," reigned supreme in Western medicine for two thousand years. In the seventeenth century, the French mathematician and philosopher René Descartes recast the animal spirits theory in terms of the mechanics that fascinated his age and led to Newton's discoveries. Descartes saw the human body as a machine, in much the same way that many today are convinced the brain functions like a computer. The human machine, according to Descartes, was powered by hydraulics, and the animal spirits that flowed through the nerves were not spirits at all but liquids. The following century was the era of discovery and experimentation with electricity, leading to the fateful day when Luigi Galvani dissected a frog on a table where he had been experimenting with static electricity, and noted that the dead frog's leg kicked when touched with a statically charged metal scalpel. Galvani concluded that the stuff that flowed through nerves was neither spirits nor fluids but electricity. "Animal spirits" were out and "animal electricity" (the new term coined by Galvani) was in.[7] The human body was revealed to be neither a house of spirits or a hydraulic machine but an electrical plant.

Whether nerves conducted spirits, fluids, or electricity, Western medicine in the eighteenth and nineteenth centuries was certain that nerves constituted the primary system for the regulation of bodily function, and "nervous disorders" dominated Western medical thinking for two hundred years. All complaints for which no lesion could be identified were thought to reside in the nervous system.[8] This covered a huge range of maladies, many of them difficult to explain in terms of what was actually known about the nervous system. In the meantime, advances in chemistry offered glimpses of the component parts of bones, blood, and tissues, which suggested that some human ailments might be based in chemistry. But what might the important chemicals be, and where did they come from? Where might one begin looking for them? With thousands of years of experience crushing and slicing the testicles of men and a variety of animals, and the extensive documentation of the behavioral and physiological changes that ensued, the obvious first place to look was the testicle.

The Birth of Endocrinology and the First Transgender Beings

Thus it was that in 1767 a Scottish surgeon named John Hunter transplanted the testicles of a rooster into the belly of a hen. Hunter did not see any change in the hen he thought was significant, so he wrote some notes for his files and forgot about it, publishing nothing about the matter.[9] A century and a half later Eugen Steinach would perform a similar experiment, find the results monumental, and set into motion a powerful chain reaction of social repercussions that continues to pick up steam today. Were the results of Hunter's and Steinach's experiments really so different, or did they see similar results through lenses of different cultural expectations? Unable to answer this question, all we can do is note that the problem of assigning meaning to the physiological effects of "sex hormones" has vexed the field of endocrinology from its first tentative beginnings.

Before moving on, we should note that, according to today's de facto definition of *transgender* (males taking estrogen and females taking testosterone), Hunter's hen with the implanted rooster testicles has the distinction of being the first documented transgender being on earth.

Nearly a hundred years after Hunter's experiment, a German physiologist, Arnold Berthold, castrated not one but six roosters. He then surgically inserted their own testicles back into the abdomens of two of the roosters and implanted two others with testicles that were not their own. The final two roosters were left testicle-less. Berthold noted that all the roosters' combs (the red fleshy growth on the rooster's head) shriveled after castration, but grew back on birds that had been "retestified." Since the implanted testicles had been inserted into the abdomen and were not connected to the hosts' bodies by nerves, Berthold had demonstrated that some mechanism other than nerves was at play. Bodies were not just hard-wired, and nerves were not their only communication system. There was a wireless system as well, and the blood was its broadcast medium.[10] Berthold's work went virtually unnoticed, but other experiments around the same time concerning an assortment of bodily functions confirmed that "external secretions" like tears, sweat, and urine did not account for all the secretory powers of the human body. There was a system of "internal secretions" from "ductless glands" as well, though what these secretions were and how they regulated body function remained shrouded in mystery.[11]

Hysteria

What really got the "internal secretions" ball rolling was not the castration of roosters but the castration of women. Thousands upon thousands of women. The doctors who performed these surgeries did not imagine themselves to be conducting endocrinological research. They thought they were treating hysteria, a disease that was the most commonly diagnosed human ailment in Europe and the United States for two hundred years but is now thought not to exist. The history of hysteria foreshadows events in our present day, including a sudden increase in incidence of a disease that had been known long before; surgeries that were considered cutting edge at the time but barbaric by later standards; the close interplay of disease, belief, and what we now call identity; the limits of scientific knowledge; the role of profit in medicine; and more. So it is worth our while to detour through the history of this remarkable disease.

As we've seen, ancient medicine located the root of femininity not in the ovaries but in the uterus. Ancient Greek medicine accordingly attributed many female afflictions to the uterus, and the term *hysteria* comes from the Greek word for uterus. The Greeks believed that the uterus, when engorged by accumulated fluid, would tear loose from its moorings and wander through the body causing a wide assortment of problems and disease, including a sense of choking, loss of speech, and depriving "the patient of all sensibility, in the same manner as if she had fallen in epilepsia." The second-century Roman doctor Galen, whose intellectual legacy dominated Western medical thought for over a thousand years, disputed that the uterus could wander but affirmed that hysteria was a uterine disease. In Galen's opinion, the cause was sexual deprivation (which caused fluid to accumulate) and sexual intercourse the cure.[12] A millennium and a half after Galen, not much had changed. The seventeenth-century French physician Lazare Riviére recommended that if marriage failed as a cure, "the Genital Parts should be by a cunning Midwife so handled and rubbed, so as to cause an Evacuation of the over-abounding Sperm" (female "Sperm," that is).[13]

After having been around in some form or another for millennia, the incidence of hysteria rose markedly in tandem with the rise of the capitalist bourgeoisie in Europe and the United States. By the seventeenth century, one noted English doctor estimated hysteria to be "the most common of all diseases except fevers." Over the next two hundred years, the scourge grew to such epidemic proportions that by 1870 an American doctor estimated that treatment of hysteria accounted for *three-fourths of all the money Americans spent on medical care.*[14] The signature symptom was the "hysterical fit," which might proceed from sobbing to laughing, to abrupt loss of speech or hearing, trances that might last for days, convulsions, and sudden paralysis or chronic fatigue that could result in lifelong disability. One New York doctor wrote, "Let the reader imagine the patient writhing like a serpent upon the floor, rending her garments to tatters, plucking out handsful of hair, and striking her person with violence."[15] Among the nineteenth century's many high-profile hysteria victims was Florence Nightingale, the indefatigable founder of modern nursing, who after an extraordinary early career spent most of the last twenty-three years of her life confined to a couch, and completely bedridden for six of them.[16]

As the number of hysterics skyrocketed and the variety of symptoms associated with the disease proliferated, doctors debated whether so many patients with such diverse symptoms indeed suffered a single disease with a single cause, and if so what that cause might be. All agreed that hysteria was a "nervous disorder," but what was the specific nervous malfunction? Events thought to trigger the onset of hysteria included physical or emotional trauma, "overcivilization," the education of women (which was held to make women literally sick), and masturbation and sexual excess (inverting the received wisdom of the previous two thousand years, which held that sexual stimulation could *cure* the disease). The range of treatments was just as varied, including changes in diet (including forced feeding, which foreshadowed today's anorexia treatment), sexual and educational abstinence, electric shock, induced vomiting, applying leeches to the vulva or anus, applying caustics (burning agents) to the clitoris and other parts of the body, and finally the surgical removal of the clitoris to destroy the "deep-seated nerve irritation."[17]

Battey's Operation, or the Normal Ovariotomy

The introduction of effective anesthesia and antisepsis in the mid-nineteenth century made invasive surgery routine for the first time, as the pain associated with operations diminished while the chances of surviving the ordeal increased. The medical men of the era built their claim to scientific credibility on these seemingly miraculous advances, and the figure of the surgeon dominated the imagination of both medical specialists and the public. Around the same time, gynecology emerged as a medical specialty. Predictably enough, surgical removal of the ovaries (ovariotomy, today more often called oophorectomy) became a common procedure for treating gynecological disorders.[18] When some gynecologists claimed to have found a coincidence between "female lunacies" and ovarian cycles, the possibility of a surgical cure for hysteria appeared on the horizon. This meeting of the magic of surgery with the epidemic of hysteria was such a no-brainer that the surgical removal of ovaries to treat hysteria was independently introduced in Germany, England, and the United States within days of each other in 1872. The surgeons called the procedure a "normal ovariotomy" because the ovaries being removed were not diseased but "normal." In the United States it was known as "Battey's Operation" after Robert Battey, an American surgeon from Rome (Rome, Georgia, that is) who proselytized more loudly than anyone in its favor.

Even with the advances in the safety of surgery, the initial death rate for "normal ovariotomy" patients was a *third* of all patients treated. After a decade of experience, that number fell and a "veritable mania for ovariotomy" swept the United States and to a lesser extent Britain and Europe.[19] The operations were deemed so successful that soon normal ovariotomies were performed to treat not only hysteria but "all cases of lunacy." One psychiatric hospital installed an annex for the sole purpose of removing ovaries from female patients, though the large majority of surgeries were performed on patients whose "female lunacies" were not severe enough to require psychiatric hospitalization. To the contrary, as news of the surgery's alleged success spread, women besieged doctors begging for the operation. There is no way to know how many women lost their ovaries in this manner, but the high-end estimates put the total at over 100,000.[20]

Bitter controversy within the medical profession surrounded these procedures. To those who championed them, they were "one of the unequalled triumphs of surgery," and those who wanted to keep them from women who desperately demanded them were "wanting in humanity" and "guilty of criminal neglect of patients." There was a sense of national pride in countries where the largest number of normal ovariotomies were performed, much as countries today compete to be at the cutting edge of stem cell research. Critics of the procedure were just as adamant, casting the surgeons performing the operations as "gynaecological perverts" whose "evil and uselessness cannot be too strongly condemned." One doctor even performed a placebo surgery as a form of criticism by simply making an incision and sewing it back up, then widely reporting his placebo "cure." One of the procedure's loudest supporters countered by announcing that the same patient had come to him a year later suffering from incessant vomiting, which he had cured by actually removing the ovaries.[21]

One of the ironies of these surgeries, which today are regarded as one of the biggest catastrophes of modern medicine, was that they resulted in a sudden increase in medical knowledge concerning the ovary. Men had been castrated by the thousands and for thousands of years, but not women. Today, bilateral oophorectomies are thought to increase the long-term risk for a number of diseases, but the doctors who performed Battey's Operation could not have known this. Indeed, in the late nineteenth century knowledge of the ovary was so crude that surgeons performing Battey's Operation were surprised when removal of the ovaries led to amenorrhea (absence of menstruation).[22] Alfred Hegar, the surgeon who first performed the procedure in Germany, insisted that women could still become pregnant after their ovaries were removed. But after thousands of oophorectomies, women who had lost their ovaries in the treatment of hysteria routinely returned to the hospital with complaints that would now be understood as severe menopausal symptoms, which tend to be more pronounced after surgically induced menopause. One result was that ovarian extracts became a common prescription for trying to alleviate the discomforts of menopause.[23] More broadly, the surgeries focused medical attention on the question of the how the gonads (ovaries in women and testicles in men) actually work.

By the turn of the century, the normal ovariotomy had fallen into disfavor amidst abundant evidence that the procedure was not merely useless but actually made the symptoms it purported to treat much worse. Robert Battey fell from the status of medical pioneer to "the destroyer of everything that makes a woman's life worth living."[24] That it took tens of thousands of surgeries over two decades to demonstrate the inefficacy of a procedure that for most of that period was thought to be almost miraculously effective was a harbinger of things to come in the field of "sex hormone" therapies.

Rejuvenation and Organotherapy

Even as Battey's star burned out, an even brighter star burst forth, promising even more dramatic results and ratcheting both medical and popular interest in the gonads up another notch. The star this time was hardly an unknown doctor from Rome, Georgia, but one of the biggest names in medicine working in Paris, France. Charles-Édouard Brown-Séquard, a physiologist and neurologist whose rapid rise took him first to the National Hospital for the Paralysed and Epileptic in London, then across the Atlantic where he was appointed professor of physiology and neuropathology at Harvard, then to Paris as professor of experimental medicine in the Collège de France. He published some five hundred essays, lectures, and journal articles. At age thirty-three he described a form of paralysis that to this day bears his name, Brown-Séquard syndrome, but his major work was on the "internal secretions." His 1856 study on adrenal glands in animals was a milestone in the nascent field of endocrinology. In addition to the testes, his research included the secretions of the thyroid, adrenal, pancreas, liver, spleen, and kidneys.[25]

So it was big news in 1889 when the magisterial seventy-two-year-old announced to a stunned audience in Paris that he had "rejuvenated" himself through self-administered "subcutaneous injections of a liquid containing a very small quantity of water mixed with the three following parts: first, blood of the testicular veins; secondly, semen; and thirdly, juice extracted from a testicle, crushed immediately after it has been taken from a dog or a guinea-pig." As a result, he reported that "a radical change took place, . . . [as I] regained at least all the strength I possessed a good many years ago." And he had hard data to back up his claims, for he had kept measurements of the strength of his arms, "the average length of the jet of urine" when he urinated, and the "power of the explosion of fecal matter" when he moved his bowels. He also noted that there were "good reasons to think that subcutaneous injections of a fluid obtained by crushing ovaries just extracted from young or adult animals, and mixed with a certain amount of water, would act on old women in a manner analogous to that of the solution extracted from the testicles injected into old men."[26]

In effect, Brown-Séquard was attempting what would become known much later as hormone replacement therapy, trying to replace the attenuated "internal secretions" of his aging glands with similar secretions extracted from young animals. Since whatever it was that testes secreted had not been identified, he figured that if he included testicular tissue *and* semen *and* blood in his concoction, he was bound to get the good stuff, whatever it might be.

To stimulate additional research concerning his revolutionary discovery, Brown-Séquard prepared more extracts to his specifications (the testicles, for example, had to be "absolutely fresh, having just been taken from the animals") and distributed them free of charge to physicians willing to test them on their patients and report back to him with the results. Other doctors quickly reported that they had repeated the experiment with equally impressive outcomes, and the gold rush was on.[27]

Soon twelve thousand doctors were administering extracts similar to Brown-Séquard's (and thousands of animals were losing their testicles).[28] "Organotherapy," or simply the "Brown-Séquard method," became a medical fad, as organs of all sorts were excised, sliced, diced, and crushed in the hopes of extracting some active ingredient that would cure some disease: thyroid was used to treat hypothyroidism; brains for neurasthenia (a spin-off diagnosis from the hysteria epidemic); pancreas for diabetes; kidney for uremia; muscle for muscular atrophy; heart for heart disease. Testicles kept their pride of place, however, with testicular extracts administered for debility, epilepsy, cancer, cholera, tuberculosis, leprosy, asthma, and more.[29] As late as 1920, the *Journal of the American Medical Association* reported that the results of "testicle organotherapy" in children "indicate that it has a tonic and stimulating influence, especially at puberty," foreshadowing by nearly a hundred years the contemporary use of hormone blockers in children diagnosed with Gender Identity Disorder (now called Gender Dysphoria).[30]

Brown-Séquard was ridiculed by many of his peers. This was the era in which the medical profession was striving to establish its scientific credentials. Since many of the common medical practices of the time were ineffectual and hardly different from folk medicine, physicians wishing to cloak themselves with the mantle of science were especially keen to draw distinctions between "scientific" medicine and folk beliefs, between "physicians" and "quacks." The Dutch Society against Quackery had been established in 1880 for just this purpose, and soon boasted more than eleven hundred members. That a physician whose "scientific" work had been hailed as second to none would fall into "quackery," and in the process spawn an entire industry of thousands of rejuvenation doctors who had none of his learned credentials, vexed these physicians to no end, but they did not have to put up with him for long. Within a few years the failure of Brown-Séquard's rejuvenation became painfully obvious, and in 1894, just five years after his alleged rejuvenation, he died at the age of seventy-seven.

As crazy as all of this sounds in hindsight, in historical context it was not as far-fetched as one might think. Just two years after Brown-Séquard's bombshell, myxedema and cretinism (congenital hypothyroidism) were traced to thyroid malfunction, and treatment of both conditions by thyroid extract, either ingested or injected, proved efficacious.[31] These were spectacular results in an age when doctors had precious few effective drugs in their tool kits, and these treatments were understood to be part of the new practice of organotherapy. Two years after that, extracts of the adrenal gland were used to successfully treat low blood pressure. (This was stumbled on by a British physician who experimented with gland extracts by feeding them to his young son.)[32] Pituitary malfunction was shown to be connected to gigantism, and surgical removal of the pancreas was shown to elevate blood sugar. Many saw all this as a vindication of Brown-Séquard's ideas.[33] A few years later, in 1922, researchers walked into a large ward of dying children in diabetic comas and began injecting them with an extract from an ox pancreas. Before they were even finished the first children to be injected were waking up. The discovery of insulin was as close to a "miracle cure" as human experience has come.[34]

"The question of the biological basis of homosexuality has been definitively solved."

In 1905, Ernest Starling coined the term *hormone* (from a Greek verb meaning "to excite or arouse") to refer to all internal secretions that regulated bodily function, and the boundaries of what would soon be called the field of endocrinology began to take shape. But though testicle research had been the nascent field's seminal event, the Brown-Séquard fiasco had cast a pronounced chill on testicle research, which subsequently languished while other organs moved to the front of the line. It would take a physician of unusual self-confidence to rehabilitate the testicle, a man like Eugen Steinach.

In 1912, Steinach set up a lab in Vienna and began intensive research on ovaries, testicles, and the hormones they were thought to secrete. Vienna was the hot spot for European experimental medicine at the time. Sigmund Freud was there, working out the theories that would soon revolutionize Western psychiatry and indeed Western culture. Josef Halban was there, too. In 1897 Halban had removed newborn guinea pig ovaries and replanted them under the skin. The guinea pigs' reproductive organs developed normally, demonstrating that ovaries, like testicles, worked their magic through the blood, and also that their secretions played a key role in early female development. Steinach's lab, officially the Institute for Experimental Biology but better known as the Vivarium, was located in the former animal house of Vienna's amusement park. It was the ideal platform for an ambitious man who hoped to make his mark at a time when physicians enjoyed enormous cultural prestige and their presentations and lectures bordered on theater.[35]

Steinach mounted an extraordinary series of experiments in the amusement park. He injected extracts of testicles, spinal cords, and brains into castrated frogs. He fed the testicular tissue of freshly killed rats to infant rats. He attempted forty-four testicular transplants on rats. He transplanted ovaries into castrated males, and testes into castrated females. Finally, he transplanted both ovaries and testes into the same rodent.

He reported that when ovaries were transplanted into castrated male rats, the bone structure, penis size, fur, and nipples all "feminized," while testicle transplants "masculinized" female rats, and that in some ways the feminized males were sometimes "hyperfeminized." He reported that the transplants determined "masculine" and "feminine" *behavior* as well. Castrated male rats with implanted ovaries exhibited what Steinach took to be characteristically female mating behavior, while females with testicles exhibited what he alleged was characteristically male mating behavior. The sexual behavior of rats with both ovaries and testicles, he claimed, was both masculine and feminine.[36]

The grand theory that Steinach spun from all of this was his theory of *sex hormone antagonism,* according to which the secretions of the testes both stimulated male sex characteristics and inhibited female character-

istics, and the secretions of the ovaries both stimulated female sex characteristics and inhibited male characteristics. He painted a portrait of a
chemical "battle" of "sharp antagonisms between masculinity and femininity." He described transplanting both ovaries and testes into the same
animal as an experiment in which male and female chemicals would be
"forced to battle it out."[37]

Steinach's work was devastatingly criticized by Carl R. Moore, an
American embryologist who attempted to repeat Steinach's experiments. Moore found that the changes Steinach interpreted as markers
of rat "feminization" and "masculinization"—body height and length,
hair structure, mammary glands, and so on—varied so widely between
individual rats that they did not reliably correlate with sex. For example, Steinach placed great importance on the increased weight of
female rats with testicle implants. Moore countered that if Steinach
had looked at a larger sample of unaltered rats he would have found
plenty of females that were larger than males. He noted that the weight
increases Steinach reported were tiny, and anyway why would a barely
measurable increase in weight be considered "masculinization" instead
of just growth?

Moore's critique of Steinach's claims about behavior was even sharper:
"Steinach has described the docility of the normal female rat (does not
fight, is easily handled, not so apt to bite or to resist handling, etc.)
but here again the variations are too great to be of any practical value.
Many females of this [i.e., Moore's] colony are decidedly more pugna-
cious than males. In several cases, these, after repeated handling, would
bite, scratch, and resemble anything other than a meek and mild-tem-
pered female of the colony."[38] With Moore's publication, a debate over
the relation between the secretions of gonads and gendered behavior was
engaged. It continues unresolved today.

As riveting as Steinach's claims about appearance and aggression
were, his claims about sexual behavior were what won him fame. To
perform sexual intercourse, one rat must expose its rump (a posture
called "lordosis") to another who must mount. Steinach claimed that
his "feminized" male rats exposed their rumps more than other males,
while "masculinized" female rats mounted more often, and concluded
that this behavior proved that human homosexuality was determined by
a pathology of the gonads.

This research unleashed a century of rat experiments that continue unabated today.[39] It turns out that female rats routinely mount both females and males, and male rats routinely expose their rumps to both males and females. Many factors affect the frequency of these behaviors, including how the rats have been socialized, their environment, stress, diet, and more. And then there is the anthropomorphism inherent in the assertion that there is a direct equivalency between rat rump-exposing and human homosexuality. It was only recently discovered that testosterone causes rat vaginas to partially close, making penetration painful. So does the reluctance of a female rat on testosterone to allow mounting constitute "homosexuality" or simply an avoidance of pain? But as far as Steinach was concerned, his gonad transplants in humping and rumping rats proved that human homosexuality was beyond all doubt a simple gonad malfunction. He even claimed he could reliably distinguish "periodic attacks" of human male homosexuality (caused by testicles that alternately produced "male" and "female" hormones) from "constant homosexuality" in humans (caused by testicles that had completely degenerated into female gonads).[40]

And so in 1919 Eugen Steinach declared to the world that "the question of the biological basis of homosexuality has been definitively solved."[41]

As with Brown-Séquard's claims a few decades before, Steinach's conceptual leap from rat gonad transplants to human homosexuality made a good fit with the assumptions of the medical milieu in which he was working. There was a new disease paradigm coming into view. Dubbed the "New Physiology," it held that each gland in the body secreted one hormone, each hormone regulated one bodily function, and a specific disease resulted when each gland produced too much or too little of its assigned hormone. Steinach's work was understood as providing experimental evidence proving the long-intuited hunch that the testicles secreted a "male sex hormone" and the ovaries secreted a "female sex hormone," and that these substances were what made men men and women women. And when European doctors in 1919 asked themselves what common and horrible disease might result from "sex hormone" deficiency, homosexuality (specifically male homosexuality) was the first thing that came to mind.

Magnus Hirschfeld and "Sexual Science"

Steinach developed his thinking on human sexuality in part through his relationship with Magnus Hirschfeld, a German-born physician. Hirschfeld was a "sexologist" at a time when men of science were first trying to extend their dominion to include human sexual behavior and desire. Hirschfeld was not the first sexologist, but he had the highest public profile, largely due to his tireless advocacy of homosexual rights. He was homosexual himself, though this was not generally known until after his death. He was the founder of the Scientific-Humanitarian Committee, the first homosexual rights organization of the modern era, and later of the Institute for Sexual Science in Berlin, which offered counseling for sexual and marital problems and advocated for sex education, contraception, treatment of sexually transmitted diseases, and women's emancipation, in addition to gaining an international reputation for its advocacy of civil rights and social acceptance for homosexuals, transexuals, and transvestites (more on Hirschfeld's taxonomy of sexual minorities later). At the time, Berlin was a magnet for homosexuals and sexual "deviants" of all types. His institute was a huge success, visited by some twenty thousand people a year until the Nazis sacked it in 1933.

Like many of today's LGBT activists, Hirschfeld believed that the public would be more tolerant of sexual minorities if they could be convinced that the cause of homosexuality lay not in any choice, life experience, or moral failing, but in something written indelibly into the body and thus beyond the reach of willpower, parenting, punishment, or prayer. And just as today's LGBT activists live in the era of the genome, Hirschfeld lived in the era of the "internal secretion" and sought the somatic source of sexual deviance in the "New Physiology" of hormones. Hirschfeld in turn was heir to the work of the pioneering homosexual rights activist Karl Heinrich Ulrichs, who died in 1895, before the age of hormones, and attributed homosexuality to the "germs" on which the scientific gaze of his time was focused. Ulrichs argued that there was "female germ" and a "male germ," and that a homosexual man was one in whom the male germ had seized control of "physical" development while the female germ had dominated the "non-physical," resulting in a "female soul in a male body."[42]

It is striking that Ulrichs and Hirschfeld, considered the first homosexual rights advocates in the modern era, were also the first to propose that homosexuality had an immediate biological cause. And that the first organized group to advocate for homosexual rights was the Scientific-Humanitarian Committee, run out of the Institute for Sexual Science, under the motto "Justice through Science." All of which suggests a deeper connection between modern sexual identities and beliefs about science than is commonly understood. While it is true that the veneer of "science" gave Hirschfeld and others a political space for homosexual advocacy that might not have been available otherwise, they were not just using "science" as a political cover. They deeply believed in their claims, and these beliefs had consequences.[43]

At the center of Hirschfeld's thinking, and indeed at the center of nearly every one of his many books, lectures, essays, and pamphlets, was his "principle of universal sexual intermediacy," by which he meant that "male" and "female" should be understood not to refer to actual people but to the far ends of a spectrum of possibility: every real person was an "intermediate" type somewhere between these extremes. Hirschfeld believed the spectrum was the result of developmental processes in the body that determined both physiology and psyche, and thus that homosexuals could be identified by physical as well as mental characteristics. Indeed, in 1903 he declared that "of the fifteen hundred homosexuals I have seen, each was physically and mentally distinct from a complete male."[44] (What an interesting specialty this secretly homosexual doctor had created for himself, requiring as it did the close examination of fifteen hundred homosexual men! Can we assume he examined an equal number of "complete males" to establish a benchmark by which to declare the homosexual body different and incomplete?) Among Hirschfeld's telltale physical manifestations of male homosexuality were limp wrists, high voices, and lack of body hair. He even claimed that homosexual men menstruated every twenty-eight days through bleeding from the mouth, nose, or anus.[45]

Hirschfeld's assertion that male homosexuals were by nature effeminate was intensely opposed by some within the Scientific-Humanitarian Committee itself, who argued that male-male love was neither a sign of femininity nor a medical pathology but an exalted form of hypermasculinity they traced back to Greek antiquity. The dissidents split from the Scientific-Humanitarian Committee to form the Union for Male Culture. The two camps detested each other, as the existence of each appeared to undermine the claims of the other.[46] How to explain the existence of big, hairy, muscular, "gender normative" male homosexuals has vexed Hirschfeld's intellectual heirs down to the present day.

Hirschfeld had been arguing since 1896 that homosexuality was a biologically determined malformation, like a harelip or cleft palate. Like Ulrichs before him, he was convinced that this made homosexuality "natural" and thus neither a criminal nor moral issue. But he could not point to the place in the body that was the source of the malformation. In 1916 he read of Richard Goldschmidt's research crossbreeding moths and butterflies. Goldschmidt claimed that his findings suggested that male human homosexuals are genetically female and vice versa. Soon Hirschfeld had a butterfly breeding operation at his institute.[47] But he lost interest in butterfly chromosomes when he heard of Steinach's work at the Vivarium, and as soon as he could he traveled to Vienna to visit Steinach and his rodents. After the visit each man began citing the other in his publications.[48] In Steinach, Hirschfeld found a star scientist whose theory of chemical bearers of gender battling it out for control of the body grounded Hirschfeld's theory of "sexual indeterminacy" on the cutting edge of experimental science. In Hirschfeld, Steinach found an indefatigable popularizer with an institute, a journal, a large client base, a busy international speaking schedule, and a mission.

Curing Male Homosexuality

Proceeding from his "proof" that homosexuality was a hormone deficiency disease, Steinach suggested that its male variant could be "cured" by transplanting properly functioning testicles into the scrotums of homosexual men. This left Hirschfeld in a bind. He had been arguing for decades that homosexuality was not a moral failing but a medical disorder, and he had publicly championed Steinach's research. Now that an effective cure for the malady seemed within reach, on what grounds could he deny such treatment to the afflicted? Finding none, Hirschfeld referred patients to Steinach for surgery, covered the surgeries in his journal, and even examined testicular tissue surgically removed from homosexuals.[49]

Steinach's first patient was a thirty-one-year-old homosexual man whose testicles had to be removed anyway due to tuberculosis, while the donor was a "normal" man whose undescended testicle also required removal. The surgery was performed by one of Steinach's colleagues. Steinach reported the surgery an unequivocal success: twelve days post-op the patient claimed to have had heterosexual erotic dreams, which were followed by sex with a female prostitute, followed by more and more sex with female prostitutes. His voice allegedly deepened and his body "masculinized." He married, and wrote to Steinach, "My wife is very satisfied with me. I am disgusted to think of the time when I felt that other passion."[50] More surgeries on homosexuals followed. Soon Steinach announced that post-op examination of the excised homosexual testicles revealed the presence of female tissue, which he dubbed "F-cells." The lesion that caused homosexuality was at long last identified.

Steinach's results were debated in the major medical forums of Europe and the United States, leading surgeons on both continents to attempt to replicate his results. It is difficult to reconstruct how many surgeries took place, but surgeries were certainly done in Vienna, London, New York, and Chicago. One surgeon who had begun as a Steinach supporter even transplanted a testicle from a "genuine homosexual" into a heterosexual man but reported that no homosexual behavior resulted. No other surgeon, however, was able to replicate Steinach's success in "curing" homosexuality or in finding the alleged "F-cells."[51]

In Europe, only Hirschfeld stuck by Steinach, continuing to cite his work in support of his own theories of homosexuality for some time after. Finally Hirschfeld too lapsed into silence on the matter. That left Harry Benjamin, a German-born doctor in New York City who described himself as Steinach's disciple, as pretty much the only person in the world still championing this part of Steinach's work, and he continued to do so until his death in 1986.

"Dr. Steinach Coming to Make Old Young"

Soon Steinach himself lost interest in curing homosexual men, for he had found much more plentiful fish to fry: he would rejuvenate old men. His method was curiously simple: he would sever the vas deferens (the tube that carries sperm from the testicle to the urethra at ejaculation).

Commonly known today as a vasectomy, it requires a procedure of only thirty minutes with local anesthetic. It is currently the most widely used method of male sterilization. But sterilization requires severing the tubes from both testicles. Steinach would severe just one, leaving the patient with the ability to father a child.

Steinach claimed his vasectomies changed the relative proportion of cells in the testicle in a way that would "rejuvenate" the patient: the germinal cells would atrophy, leaving more space for the Leydig cells—the cells that produce testosterone, first discovered in 1850, although their exact function was still unclear—to proliferate, which would lead to increased production of "male sex hormone," which would replenish the recipient with the vigor of youth. While few nonspecialists could follow Steinach's argument about the cells of the testicle, the idea that one could conserve manhood by ejaculating semen back into the body rather than scattering one's seed hither and yon in the big wide world was intuitive. This was, after all, an era obsessed with the fear that masturbation led to disease, insanity, and loss of manhood. And once again Steinach had more rat experiments to back him up, reporting that the old, nearly lifeless rats subjected to the procedure gained weight, glossy new fur, and sexual desire, with some having intercourse nineteen times in fifteen minutes.[52]

The first human surgery was performed in 1918 on a forty-three-year-old coachman who suffered from what we would now call chronic fatigue. To eliminate the effect of suggestion, the procedure was done without the patient's knowledge during a surgery for other purposes. In 1920 Steinach reported the results in a book illustrated with photographs of the apparently extraordinary outcome:

> The patient presented the appearance of an exhausted and prematurely old man. His weight was 108 pounds, his musculature was weak, and there was very little cushion of fat. The skin was dull and conspicuously dry, the hair grey and had fallen out on top, scanty beard, lank hair growth on the trunk and extremities. . . . The ex-patient now drags loads of up to 220 pounds with ease. His muscles have developed extraordinarily. The hair on his head is thicker and his beard more strongly developed. The head and face hair grow so quickly he has to have it cut and shaved twice as often as previously. . . . The skin appears soft, with fine down, pliable and moist. . . . This man with his smooth, unwrinkled face, his smart and upright bearing, gives the impression of a man at the height of his vitality.[53]

A media frenzy ensued. Among the extensive coverage the *New York Times* gave the matter over the following decades was this story from 1923:

> As soon as it was certain that this was no mere comic supplement jest, and that Steinach was a real scientist, the exodus to Vienna began. Some surgeons simply dropped everything and departed; they wanted to be first on the ground and back again. Some went without ostentation; others were somewhat blatant about it. Their return was heralded in various ways. . . .
>
> [A]t this moment there is probably no city in the country large enough to support . . . a first-class practitioner of general surgery but has its quota of "Steinach rejuvenation" patients. . . .
>
> In Europe knowledge of Steinach's theories and practice is being promulgated rapidly by means of filmed reproductions of the results of surgical procedure, both on rats and on men. A cable from Vienna last week told in extravagant language that crowds were clamoring to get into the movie houses where the film was being shown, and that they stood around disconsolately when they were unable to gain admission. Aged male rats were shown barely able to stand. Next came the operation. Then followed the pictured process of rejuvenation. The rats were shown to be "young" and playful. Finally they were depicted surrounded by new offspring. The condition of a man before, during, and subject to the operation was also pictured. . . .
>
> A recent cable from Vienna said that Steinach was likely to receive the Nobel prize in medicine this year for his work in the retardation of senility in man.[54]

Steinach never won his Nobel prize, but he was nominated for it six different years.

By 1926 New York City alone had one hundred surgeons offering to "Steinach" their patients, among whom the most vocal was Steinach's tireless publicist and disciple, Harry Benjamin. As Benjamin explained in the *New York Medical Journal:* "The point that so far has not been brought out with necessary clearness is that by the Steinach operation the patient is given a more or less massive and continuous dose of his own gonadal hormone. . . . All symptoms due to senility, including sexual impotence, as a rule improve after the operation."[55]

Eventually Benjamin would perform hundreds of the procedures at his Life Extension Institute in New York, claiming the operation would "increase the productive yield of great men: scientists, inventors, artists." The poet William Butler Yeats was Steinached in London at age sixty-nine. Yeats spoke so often of his resulting "second puberty" that the Dublin press nicknamed him the "gland old man." "It revived my creative power," Yeats proclaimed. "It revived also sexual desire; and that in all likelihood will last me until I die."[56]

Nor were women without rejuvenating remedy, for Steinach declared that subjecting the ovaries to x-rays would produce the same benefits for women by altering the ratio of cells in the ovary. The American novelist Gertrude Atherton had her ovaries irradiated and then wrote her best-selling 1923 novel *Black Oxen,* the story of a man who falls in love with an Austrian countess whom he believes to be a young woman but is actually fifty-eight years old, having regained her youth through a rejuvenating glandular treatment and x-ray surgery.[57] Atheron's enthusiasm led her to suggest that Germany, having lost so many young men in the Great War, could regain its former glory "by having her supermen subjected to the Steinach treatment and rejuvenated." This was not idle talk. It is estimated that a million vasectomies were performed in the Third Reich for this purpose.[58]

Testicles: Monkey, Goat, Boar, Ram, Deer, Bull, Felon

Steinach had some stiff competition in the rejuvenation market, most notably from Serge Voronoff, a Russian physiologist working in Paris, who reasoned that if Brown-Séquard's injections of crushed animal testicles had not done the trick, perhaps testicle transplants would. Since human testicle donors were in short supply, Voronoff turned to monkeys. By 1926 he had performed one thousand surgeries grafting tissue from monkey testicles into humans.[59] He became fabulously wealthy, dividing his time between a villa on the Italian Riviera and Paris, where his living quarters occupied the entire first floor of one of the city's most expensive hotels (while his chauffeurs, valets, personal secretaries, and chefs lived on the top floor). Across the Atlantic, *Scientific American* proclaimed, "Even death, save by accident, may become unknown, if the daring experiments of Dr. Serge Voronoff, brilliant French surgeon, continue to produce results such as have startled the world."[60]

These were not fringe operators. The work of Steinach, Voronoff, and their many followers was published in the most prestigious medical journals of the day. They lectured at the most prestigious medical schools. Voronoff was invited to write an entry on rejuvenation in the *Encyclopedia Britannica.* A nationalist rejuvenation war ensued, which echoed the competition in ovariotomies to treat hysteria a few decades earlier. Germany and Austria backed Steinach, France was Voronoff country, and Britain and America leaned toward Voronoff, with the exception of Steinach's vocal champion in New York, Harry Benjamin.

The supply of monkey testicles emerged as a major concern. Voronoff set up a monkey house on the Italian Riviera run by a former circus animal keeper. In Chicago, the noted American surgeon Max Thorek, who had performed ninety-seven such operations and published a book titled *The Human Testis,* had a monkey house build on the roof of American Hospital. Both the French and Belgian governments acted to conserve the monkey supply, banning the killing of monkeys for fur in their African colonies.[61]

Voronoff was not the only testicle evangelist. An American urologist, George Frank Lydston, had done a number of human testicle transplants in 1914, including one on himself. His sober reports, claiming that the operations retarded senility and cured gray hair, psoriasis, and sexual disorders, were published in a number of medical journals.[62] John R. Brinkley set up a surgical clinic in the tiny town of Milford, Kansas, and began to rake in money transplanting goat testicles into eager human patients (goats being in far greater supply in Kansas than monkeys). Altogether, between 1912 and 1925 more than a thousand men, most of them in America, received testicular grafts from sheep, monkeys, goats, deer . . . and humans.[63]

Over the course of ten years at the San Quentin Penitentiary north of San Francisco, Leo L. Stanley routinely removed testicles from executed prisoners and implanted them in other prisoners. When the supply of executed men failed to keep up with his experiments, he began using testicles from goats, boars, rams, and deer. Stanley reported results from 643 such surgeries in the *Journal of Endocrinology,* and his work was championed by the dean of the University of California Medical School. Thanksgiving day games in the prison yard became a media spectacle of older graftees beating younger prisoners.[64]

While most of these operations aimed at rejuvenation, some continued to attempt to cure male homosexuality. Voronoff claimed a success rate of 57 percent in the treatment of "sexual inversion." In New York, H. Lyons Hunt reported curing "male perverts" with bull testicle transplants.[65] Stanley's prison surgeries addressed homosexuality in significant measure, though he left no record as to what portion of his many surgeries this amounted to. Like many of his contemporaries, Stanley believed in an endocrinological theory of crime. He linked murder and forgery with glandular defects, and mass murder with sexual ambiguity. For Stanley, curing sexual deviance and senility were one and the same endeavor, for both were symptoms of a single glandular pathology. Guilt resided primarily not in the person but the gland:

> Exhibitionism, obscene behavior, the molesting of little children, are crimes committed by the senile. This form of insanity can overtake the finest of old men, in the best of families; but why, we have yet to learn. Perhaps the outworn glands look for solace in strange directions. . . . Their condition has nothing to do with the sort of men they have been. It is due to the ghastly and humiliating processes that overwhelm weakened old humans who have outworn the procreative urge and snatch blindly at any emotion to take its place.[66]

"The Chemistry of the Soul"

Louis Berman, a Columbia University professor and cofounder of the New York Endocrinology Society, wrote a series of books on hormones that became best sellers, declaring hormones "the chemistry of the soul" and the key to unraveling the hierarchy of human race relations:

> The white man possesses more of pituitary, adrenal, gonad, and thyroid internal secretions as compared with the yellow man or the black man. And since these endocrines control not only physique and physiognomy, anatomic and functional minutiae, but also mind and behaviour, we are justified in putting down the white man's predominance on the planet to a greater all-around concentration in his blood of the omnipotent hormones.[67]

Ultimately, Berman declared that hormones promised the "chemical perfectibility of human life. . . . The chemical conditions of being are the steps of the ladder by which [man] will climb to those dizzy heights where he will stretch out his hands and find himself a God."[68] His final book, published in 1936, was titled *New Creations in Human Beings*. And right at the top of his list of things to perfect about the new humans was eradicating homosexuality.

Voronoff's surgeries ignited highly emotional public debate. Eugenicists (then at their peak of influence) warned that Voronoff's transplants might poison the "human stock" with monkey characteristics. The large and active antivivisection (or what today would be called animal rights) movement decried the mutilation of monkeys. Voronoff's suggestion that bright boys could be gland-grafted to create "a new super race of men of genius" led religious authorities and some scientists to call for a moratorium on monkey gland surgeries until the moral implications could be sorted out. This marked the first appearance in history of a demand for a moratorium on a specific line of scientific research, foreshadowing today's debates on cloning, stem cells, and other technologies. None of these critics questioned the efficacy of Voronoff's rejuvenating surgeries. Everyone agreed the surgery worked. The disagreement concerned the ethical implications of this amazing medical advance.[69]

There was no single moment when the work of Steinach, Voronoff, and the others fell from favor. Once testosterone was synthesized in the 1930s, everyone lost interest in testicles. Now that the secretions of testicles could be produced in the lab in any quantity desired, who wanted to maintain a house full of monkeys?

Voronoff's fall was precipitated not by the results of the more than one thousand testicle surgeries he personally performed on men, but from the later surgeries he performed on sheep, horses, and bulls, claiming that testicular grafts would produce results such as sheep that grew more and better wool. Unfortunately for Voronoff, sheep are not as susceptible to the power of suggestion as people. To appreciate the power of the placebo effect of Voronoff's surgeries on humans, consider that his patients were paying an enormous sum of money for a procedure they very much wanted to succeed, and whose intended outcome was hard to measure in any event. The patient would be laid out in one operating room, while a monkey was laid out in an adjoining room. The most famous surgeon in the world would then anesthetize both and work his magic. Who would return home from such an experience and not notice at least some sort of "rejuvenation"? Sheep were apparently less impressed by all this, and unlike "rejuvenation," the amount of wool a sheep produces can be precisely measured. After dazzling the top medical schools and journals for a decade, Voronoff's claims finally bit the dust in the barnyard.[70]

The Age of the Gonad

The period from the first "normal ovariotomy" in 1872 to the last testicle graft in the 1930s may be considered the age of the gonad. In Europe, the United States, and to a lesser extent worldwide, thousands upon thousands of men and women had surgery on their gonads for the purpose of altering both their physiology and behavior: to stop their hysterical fits, increase their productivity and creativity, increase their heterosexual desire and prowess, and decrease their homosexual desire. Ovaries were removed or irradiated. Testicles were snipped, removed, inserted, irradiated, transplanted, and grafted. Monkeys, rams, goats, boars, bulls, and human prisoners sacrificed their testicles to the cause. Huge fortunes were made. The surgeries were performed at the top hospitals, reported in the top medical journals, championed by the leading medical authorities, and covered in the major newspapers. The world's leading homosexual rights champion endorsed these efforts.

By the second half of the twentieth century, all of these surgeries were understood to have had either negative effects or no effect at all. Millions of men have vasectomies as birth control procedures, and none report being rejuvenated (since sterilization requires vasectomies on not one but both testicles, the rejuvenating effect of today's dual vasectomies should be twice that of a Steinach procedure). Present-day medical knowledge holds that tissue transplanted from animals to humans is quickly destroyed by the recipient's immune system unless immunosuppressant drugs are used, drugs that were not available in Voronoff's day. As noted earlier, oophorectomies are now known to cause surgically induced menopause, which can result in severe menopausal symptoms and also carries long-term health risks.

In hindsight, what is perhaps most perplexing is that throughout the age of the gonad there was never much complaint from the patients. To the contrary, they showered their surgeons with glowing reviews. In the vast majority of cases, the surgeries were eagerly sought out by the patients, who would pay almost any fee. In the case of normal ovariotomies, women would go from doctor to doctor begging for the operation, accusing those who refused them of medical neglect.

Given his position in Paris and the flamboyance of both his procedure and his character, Voronoff's fall was spectacular. By the time of his death in 1951, he had become an iconic medical laughingstock. The reputation of Steinach, who never could match Voronoff's unerring instinct for publicity and was forced into exile by the Nazis, suffered a more gradual decline. He is remembered today more as a tragedy than a farce, a scientist whose research went hopelessly wrong. But David Hamilton, a surgeon and historian who wrote the only book-length investigation of these matters, argues that this judgment is upside down. Hamilton points out that Voronoff invited more scrutiny of his work than Steinach would allow, and seems to have reported results he honestly thought were valid. Steinach reported on faked experiments, and one of his assistants eventually committed suicide just days after being accused of secretly injecting ink into a frog specimen to make it appear to support his conclusions.[71]

The medical world has done its best to forget about all of it. Steinach's 1944 obituary in the *New York Times*—the newspaper that had breathlessly hyped his research for so many years—claimed that "physicians never took him too seriously."[72] Only diehard Harry Benjamin remained faithfully at his master's side, writing to the *Times* that he still considered himself a Steinach "disciple," and that "the theory by which he explained his results which were undoubtedly achieved gave rise to scientific arguments which are not yet settled."[73]

The reader may be surprised to learn that of all these men, the two whose legacies are most alive and kicking, far more influential in death than they were in life, are Harry Benjamin and John R. Brinkley, the Kansas surgeon whose specialty was transplanting goat testicles.

Brinkley was ultimately barred from medical practice in Kansas, not for performing useless surgeries but for faking his medical credentials, and is generally remembered as a huckster and swindler who did not believe in the efficacy of his own surgeries. Yet he can just as easily be understood as smart guy who realized that there are medical procedures that "work" because people believe they work, so why not give people what they want? Seen in this light, his legacy casts a longer shadow in today's medical world than many of his contemporaries. Brinkley responded to his banishment from medical practice in Kansas by using his high-wattage radio station (which he had built to promote his surgeries) to back a run for state governor, which he very nearly won despite being a late-entry write-in candidate. In his innovative use of media for an end-run around medical authorities to appeal directly to a motivated patient base, Brinkley foreshadowed the role of the Internet and direct-to-consumer prescription medicine advertising in today's "client-centered medicine."

Harry Benjamin went on to become the founder of today's transgender health care. Until 2007, the world's principle international advocacy organization for trans health care, the World Professional Organization for Transgender Health, was named the Harry Benjamin International Gender Dysphoria Association. It confers a yearly Harry Benjamin Lifetime Distinguished Scientific Achievement Award, and promotes a set of clinical guidelines for the treatment of the transgendered, originally called the Harry Benjamin Standards of Care.

2

The "Male Sex Hormone" and the Testosterone Gold Rush

With all the hubbub over organotherapy on the one hand, and major advances in the tools and basics of chemistry on the other, it was obvious that if "sex hormones" could be chemically identified and isolated, perhaps the chemicals themselves, rather than the testicles and ovaries that produced them, could be harvested from animals. Even better, perhaps the chemicals could be synthesized in a lab more cheaply than they could be harvested. No one knew exactly what these substances would be useful for, but many were certain they would be good for *a lot.* Thus the beginning of the twentieth century saw the first big chemical-pharmaceutical gold rush, with major enterprises in several countries racing to be the first to patent a "sex hormone." Chemistry seemed to teeter on the brink of alchemy, with all sights fixed on a compound that would, like the philosopher's stone of legend, extend life and turn everything to gold. The race produced not only the first pharmaceutical hormones but also the giant pharmaceutical corporations that continue to dominate the world drug market to this day.

"Male sex hormones" and "female sex hormones" remained hypothetical substances. The *idea* that they existed resulted from the intersection of the ancient belief that testicles were the source of manhood, the comparatively recent belief that ovaries were the source of womanhood, and the "New Physiology," which asserted that each endocrine gland secreted one hormone with one function. It followed that the one thing testicles produced was the "male sex hormone," and the one thing ovaries produced was the "female sex hormone."

The first question confronting those prospecting for hormone gold was this: How would they know when they had found it? In the sex hormone sweepstakes, how would a contestant be judged the winner? It was an unusual question. This research did not involve finding something in the body and then trying to figure out how it worked. Rather, researchers were imagining something they felt certain must be there, and then trying to find it.

The idea was to castrate lab animals and observe the physiological changes that ensued. If a substance could be developed that reversed the changes observed in the castrated animal, the discovery of a "sex hormone" would be declared. After a lot of debate and false starts, it was agreed that the standard for the "male sex hormone" would be the size of a rooster's comb. When a rooster is castrated its comb shrinks. Whoever found a substance that would make a castrated rooster's comb grow back would be judged to have found the "male sex hormone." Potency was to be measured by how fast the comb grew back and to what size. This standard had the advantage that the rooster did not have to be killed and dissected to determine the outcome, so the same bird could be used again and again. Researchers didn't even need a microscope, as the comb was plainly visible.

For the "female sex hormone," it was likewise judged that the standard should be some aspect of the body that changed as a result of oophorectomy, which the sought-after substance should return to its original state. The first candidate for the standard was uterus weight, since the uterus had been considered the source of femininity since ancient times. But weighing a uterus required killing and dissecting the animal, which was costly and time consuming. Behavioral tests were proposed, but no one could agree on how to measure the femininity of behavior. (Steinach thought measuring feminine behavior was a slam dunk, but then he had his Vivarium all to himself and did not have to trouble himself with competitors trying to make similar measurements. In the twenty-first century, measuring the femininity of behavior would become a staple of sex hormone endocrinology, but we are getting ahead of the story.) At one point "female sex hormone" potency was measured in two competing rat units, a mouse unit, and an "international unit." Finally everyone settled on a vaginal smear for mice, to test for cornification (an enlarging and flattening of certain cells) in the vaginal wall related to the estrous cycle.[1]

Efforts continued on a smaller scale to test whether candidate substances could cure homosexuality, on the assumption that homosexuality was the result of "sex hormone" deficiency and thus that anything that cured it must indeed be the sought after "sex hormone." For one glorious moment, homosexuality was measured in mouse and rooster units.

To enter the race, contestants had to secure access to enormous amounts of human or animal parts or waste to sift through, looking for stuff that would cornify the vaginal wall of a mouse or make a rooster's comb grow. Researchers collected animal gonads from slaughterhouses and human testicles from executed prisoners. British chemists managed to get hold of the gigantic ovaries of a blue whale. Chemists in Berlin collected 25,000 liters of policemen's urine. Dutch researchers received delivery of an entire trainload of tanker cars filled with nothing but horse urine.[2]

Almost immediately, however, things got confusing. In 1921 came a report that extracts of mouse testicles made mouse uteruses grow, just like ovary extracts did. Six years later came the discovery that the "female sex hormone" was present in the testes and urine of men. Not homosexual men, as the scientists reporting the discovery were at pains to make clear, but "normal healthy men." In 1934 horse testicles were discovered to have more "female sex hormone" than any other tissue on earth. And while mares had small amounts of "female sex hormone" in their urine, stallion piss was loaded with it—one hundred to two hundred times that of a mare.[3] In other words, whatever was in stallion urine was as much as two hundred times better at cornifying the walls of mouse vaginas than whatever was in mare urine. Not even pregnant mares could compete with that icon of male virility, the stallion, in terms of chemical femininity. Given some urine from an unknown horse, a chemist could easily identify its sex: if the piss was loaded with "female sex hormone," the horse was a stud.

The papers that reported these findings were strewn with phrases like "surprising observations," "strange and apparently anomalous discoveries," and "paradoxical findings." One researcher felt compelled to emphasize that the urine he had worked with came from men whose "masculine character and ability to impregnate females" were well established. Others concluded that the problem must result from unknown sex pathologies in their test subjects, whom they labeled "latent hermaphrodites." But as chemists isolated substances that could potently grow a rooster comb and cornify a mouse vagina, these were definitively shown to be present in men and women of all shapes, sizes, and proclivities.[4]

For a moment these disquieting facts seemed to threaten the whole scientific edifice of gender. How can men have within them the "essence" of women, and women the "essence" of men? What were these things *doing* in there? One theory was that they were causing disease, particularly homosexuality. Others proposed an updating of Steinach's old "antagonism" thesis: the chemicals were battling it out for gender control. The day was saved by *gender spectrum theory,* in effect an update of Hirschfeld's old "principle of universal sexual intermediacy." The idea here was to replace the notion that male hormones make men and female hormones make women with the idea that gender is created by different *ratios* of male and female hormones. Actual people were said to exist not as "men" or "women" but along a spectrum of differing ratios of chemicals, resulting in a range that went from manly men to effeminate men to manly women to effeminate women. The rigid binary of male and female chemicals was rescued by sacrificing the rigid gender binary of people. People were no longer clearly male or female, but chemicals were.

Of course, if these chemicals had not been hypothesized as "male" and "female" in the first place, all of these theoretical contortions would have been unnecessary. The fact that the same chemicals circulate in both male and female bodies would not have threatened anything, and manhood and womanhood would have emerged unscathed.

Then it was discovered that the ovaries produce not one "female sex hormone" but two, and then three.

The one gland / one hormone model came crashing down. Then the liver and adrenal glands were found to produce the same stuff. Then the adrenal gland was found to secrete "male sex hormones" as well. There was talk of designating the adrenal gland the "third male gonad." Researchers reported that when the adrenal glands of boys were surgically removed, "cases of homosexuality have undergone a subtle change to normal heterosexuality." But this was followed by a study showing what seemed like the opposite, that suppression of the adrenal glands in post-pubertal males led to "feminization." A discussion of the "undoubtedly remarkable . . . obvious bisexuality" of the adrenal gland ensued. "Adrenal virilization" in women became a major new worry. At Columbia University, Louis Berman asserted that maladjusted "adrenal types" had led the fight for woman suffrage, and warned that women with even mildly hyperfunctioning adrenal glands were "the ones who, in the present overturn of the traditional sex relationships, will become the professional politicians, bankers, captains of industry, and directors of affairs in general."[5]

Today there are thought to be three major naturally occurring estrogens in women (estrone, estradiol, and estriol) and six androgens (testosterone, dehydroepiandrosterone, androstenedione, androstenediol, androsterone, and dihydrotestosterone). Popularly we still lump the "female sex hormones" together as "estrogen" and the "male sex hormones" together as "testosterone," but this creates an apples-and-oranges confusion. "Estrogen" now refers to a class of chemicals, none of which is actually named "estrogen." "Testosterone" refers to one chemical within a class called "androgens." To make things more confusing still, all three estrogens in women's bodies are synthesized from androgens by the chemical factories we call cells. And when estrogens are metabolized, they are metabolized back to androgens. And then there are the synthetic "estrogens," which win their titles not because their chemical structures are similar to anything produced in anyone's body but because their effects on the body mimic the effects of biological estrogens.

It was only in 1958 that "the" estrogen receptor was found. (Hormones circulating in the blood lock to receptors like two pieces of a jigsaw puzzle, which then triggers a response in bodily function.) A half century passed before researchers were stunned to find a second estrogen receptor. Today it is thought that the whole system regulating "secondary sexual characteristics" involves not just gonads but many other glands and also the brain, in an exceedingly complex system of multiple feedback loops about which much is yet to be understood. We have come a long, long way from 1939, when the first textbook on sex endocrinology stated: "Sex characteristics in general are subject to certain simple mechanisms of control . . . which determine whether male or female characters shall develop in an individual. . . . The mechanisms of control are exceedingly simple. . . . As there are two sets of sex characters, so there are two sex hormones."[6]

The Isolation and Synthesis of the "Male Sex Hormone"

Though the testicles of Arnold Berthold's rooster were the first glands subjected to what we now call endocrinological research, it took nearly a century, from 1848 to 1931, to isolate and identify the testicle's secretion. This contrasts with other glands whose secretions were pursued much later yet isolated much faster. In part this was because testicles produce their secretions in such tiny amounts. Chemists struggled to secure enough raw material to sift through. While ovaries were regularly surgically removed from women, there was no medical practice of removing testicles. Urine was the next best option, but where to get it? Drug companies frantically competed to secure male urine wherever large groups of men regularly pissed: factories, barracks, police stations, and prisons. Paul de Kruif, the leading American science writer of the day, marveled, "It is as if God wished to hide testosterone from the curiosity of questing men who, if they found it, might be bold to use it to make mankind happier than God intended."[7]

At last, in 1931 a German chemist, Adolf Butenandt, purified 50 milligrams of what he called androsterone from those 25,000 liters of urine collected from Berlin policemen.[8] It was already suspected that there was *another,* more powerful "male sex hormone" secreted by the testicles, and chemists backed by pharmaceutical companies in the Netherlands, Germany, and Switzerland raced to isolate it. In 1935 they succeeded, and the substance—christened testosterone—was synthesized in the lab just a year later. Just two years after that, both testosterone propionate and methyltestosterone became commercially available.

But now the chemists encountered a completely unanticipated problem: the "male sex hormone" preparations isolated from testes and urine didn't do much of anything when administered to test subjects. Chemists from the giant Dutch firm Organon reported: "It is evident now that these preparations produce only a very moderate growth of the sexual organs in castrated infantile rats and mice, *compared to what we reasonably could have expected.* We succeeded, however, in strengthening the activity of male sex hormones . . . by means of the addition of estrone [resulting in] substances which *almost reach our ideal of a 'male hormone.'*"⁹

In other words, the mighty source of manhood secreted by the testicles didn't do much unless it was modified by the addition of the source of womanhood. "Our ideal male hormone" did not exist until chemists created it. The medical director of Organon announced the glorious feat: "Science not only introduces the synthetic production of hormones, but also constructs transformations in the molecule, in order to improve the activity of the natural substances. Evidently, man attempts to be wiser than nature itself."¹⁰

Suitably accessorized in its "feminine" attire, the chemical essence of manhood made its grand entrance onto the world stage. This was big news. Paul de Kruif proclaimed it "the most secret quintessence of life." The 1939 Nobel Prize in chemistry was awarded to the lead researchers. The Nazis had recently come to power in Germany, and the Führer himself was one of the first people to receive the wonder drug. *Business Week* declared, "Of all the sex hormones, testosterone is said to have the greatest market potential." *Time* magazine marveled that "to produce one ounce of natural testosterone would require the castration of some 1,000,000 sturdy men," and then triumphantly announced that "German and Swiss chemical laboratories are already prepared . . . to manufacture from sheep's wool all the testosterone the world needs to cure homosexuals, revitalize old men."¹¹

Curing Male Homosexuality with "Male Sex Hormones"

Sure enough, following in the footsteps of Steinach, Hirschfeld, Voronoff, and others, the first use to which "the most secret quintessence of life" was put was curing male homosexuality. The hormonal theory of homosexuality, which had been mothballed since the failure of Steinach and Voronoff treatments to "cure" it, was resurrected with a vengeance now that instead of searching for lesions in the gonads that weren't there, chemists could measure precise amounts of chemical masculinity and femininity in urine.

Clifford A. Wright, cofounder of the Psychoendocrine Clinic of the Los Angeles County General Hospital, got right to work measuring homosexual urine and reported that "the usual balance or dominance" of sex hormones "is *definitely* altered." Wright was so confident of his ability to measure human homosexuality in urine that he used "hormone assays of the urine . . . in helping to disprove homosexuality in a normal individual where arrest has been made because of an alleged overt act. The patient was a girl of seventeen, whose teacher, a homosexual woman, made love to her. The girl denied homosexual inclinations and her hormone assay was normal. Subsequent investigations confirmed these negative findings."[12]

Another group studied the urine of twenty-six "true male homosexuals" over two years and concluded that hormonal assays of homosexual urine constituted a "direct, measurable, and scientifically worthwhile approach to the sexual constitution of man."[13]

Having "proven" that homosexuality was a hormone deficiency disease, the next step was to treat the malady by administering the missing amount of the deficient chemical. It is difficult to piece together an accurate picture of how many men became victims of this, since reporting was not systematic, but the list was substantial. Wright's first patient was a twenty-four-year-old male whose mother reported that after treatment he was "interested more or less in three girls."[14] At Jewish Hospital in Cincinnati, Louis A. Lurie reported treating four adolescent boys. Echoing Hirschfeld's claim that homosexuality could be measured in hips and wrists, Lurie diagnosed these boys as having "eunuchoid skeletal development," "female skeletal development," and so on, though he summarized his diagnosis by simply asserting that "the 'fairy' is easily recognized." (At the time, "fairy" was the most widely used identifier in the homosexual subculture, though its precise meaning does not match with any term in use today.) Lurie was pleased with his results, which "were startling": "His voice became deep. . . . There was a marked change in his personality. Instead of a fearful, highly emotional and demonstrative effeminate boy, he became a pleasing type of aggressive male." As a crowning achievement, two of his teenage patients joined the armed forces.[15]

At the Delaware state mental hospital, Dr. Charles W. Dunn administered testosterone to boys between nine and thirteen years of age who, Paul de Kruif wrote, "were no good at football, baseball, and basketball, and their low mental energy kept them behind in their school work. And they were ashamed, and felt inferior. . . . Shrewdly, Dr.

Dunn brought these physically and mentally laggard boys up toward the condition of their classmates with little doses of testosterone. . . . They could play and fight. . . . They began growing pubic hair and hair under their arms. They were no longer ashamed after games when they went to the showers."[16]

Soon there were a variety of "sex hormone" products to choose from, so when one treatment failed to cure, more options were provided free of charge by drug companies eager to consolidate their position in the emerging market for curing homosexuality. In one case, over the course of six months, a "negro of the passive homosexual type" was given oral stilboestrol (a synthetic estrogen also known as DES, which we will get to know more intimately shortly), an implanted 150-milligram pellet of testosterone, shots containing a gonadotropic preparation derived from pregnant mare serum as well as injections of pituitary gonadotropic and testosterone propionate, thyroid extract to "enhance the responsivity to sex hormones," and finally Emmenin and Estriol, both estrogens. At long last his discouraged doctors reported that the only verifiable result of this cornucopia of chemicals was nausea.[17]

Curing Male Homosexuality with "Female Sex Hormones"

What ultimately rescued homosexual men from these "cures" was not any perceived lack of efficacy of the treatments but rather an increasing awareness of testosterone's power as a sexual stimulant. (If you want to hear a hearty laugh, tell a female-to-male "transman" who is shooting testosterone regularly that at one time doctors thought that such a regimen would cure male homosexuality. One such person to whom I related this history not only burst into laughter but jumped up and began merrily humping the table, the chair, the wall, and everything else within reach.)

Amping up the sex drive of homosexual men was hardly what the doctors had in mind, so the whole treatment paradigm was simply turned upside down. Beginning in the late 1940s homosexual men (usually those who had fallen into the hands of police) were treated not with testosterone but with estrogen, on the theory that since testosterone seemed to stimulate homosexual desire, estrogen might suppress it. This marked a particularly bizarre chapter in an already strange story, since male homosexuality was thought by many researchers to be the result of excess exposure to estrogens. Estrogen became male homosexuality's cause and cure.

One of the first homosexual estrogen casualties was Alan Turing, the brilliant British mathematician who played a key role in cracking the secret code used in Nazi radio transmissions during World War II, and the subject of the feature film *The Imitation Game.* Turing is today considered the founder of computer science, and the annual Turing Prize is one of the most coveted in the field. In 1952 Turing was arrested for homosexuality and sentenced to estrogen treatment. His breasts started to grow. In 1954 he committed suicide.[18] Thousands of less famous men received similar punishment. Once homosexuality was decriminalized in the United States and England, homosexual men were no longer fair game for this sort of chemical torture, but as we will see, the practice is still very much alive in other parts of the world.

None of this was discussed outside the confines of medicine and law, since in the United States it was illegal to mail anything that discussed homosexuality in print. Major newspaper reports on these treatments obliquely referred to experiments with "eunuchoid men" and the like.[19] Public discussion of testosterone focused instead on the gold to be mined from male "rejuvenation."

A Miracle Drug without a Disease

Promotional material for the first testosterone drug, dubbed Neo-Hombreol, arrived in doctors' offices in 1939, proclaiming that "proper administration of testosterone propionate can play the same role in man as does estrogen therapy in the menopause, the female climacteric." These early marketing materials for testosterone mark the first mention in any medical literature anywhere in history of a "male climacteric" alleged to be the male equivalent of female menopause. The appearance of this new disease was not prompted by a single new study on the male aging process, or by any case of a sick individual, but simply by the arrival of a new product to sell. Nevertheless, drug companies reported an "almost incredible" response: "We received more requests for free samples of Neo-Hombreol than for any pharmaceutical we have ever introduced." Doctors were apparently eagerly trying the samples out on themselves.[20]

In addition to their "rejuvenating" properties, testosterone products were touted as therapeutic for men suffering from "sexual dysfunction" and as treatment for prostate cancer.

No drug company marketing could match the impact of Paul de Kruif's 1945 book, *The Male Hormone.* De Kruif was a major force in publishing. He wrote more than a dozen books and two hundred magazine articles. His 1926 book *Microbe Hunters* sold more than a million copies and was translated into eighteen languages.[21] He pulled out all the stops in his testosterone manifesto, which was excerpted in *Reader's Digest,* reviewed in the *New York Times,* and received a full-page article in *Time* magazine.[22] De Kruif told of the heroic lives of the chemists associated with testosterone, describing one of them as "a rough-and-tumble death-fighting type" and others as "toiling with bull testicles in Chicago, . . . extracting oceans of urine in Göttingen, . . . [and] dabbling dangerously with cholesterol in Zurich." These were manly men who ate steak, drank whiskey, and with Herculean effort moved geriatrics from a "sissy science" to a medical practice of "total vitality." "Yes," de Kruif declared, "sex is chemical and the male sex chemical seemed to be the key not only to sex but to enterprise, courage, and vigor." He repeated this message again and again. "Manhood is chemical, manhood is testosterone."[23]

Hype, hype, hype, and then . . . nothing. The testosterone tsunami that was forecast to wash over Western culture failed to materialize.

Testosterone, in turned out, did not cure prostate cancer but made it worse. Oops. The promised rejuvenation was difficult to detect. Few of the doctors who tried the free samples on themselves felt sufficiently rejuvenated to order more of the stuff for their patients.[24]

Women, meanwhile, were being given testosterone for all sorts of reasons that contemporary medicine would consider absurd: surgically induced menopause, metastatic breast cancer, a variety of gynecological disorders, uterine bleeding, and more. At best testosterone had no effect on these conditions. It had been anticipated that the chemical would be sexually stimulating to men, but doctors were stunned when women too began reporting sudden eruptions of sexual desire. How could the "male sex hormone" sexually stimulate women? The women were even more startled than their doctors. The effect was often unwelcome, in part because intense sexual desire was considered unladylike at the time. And anyway, who wants a raging sex drive while suffering from metastatic breast cancer or uncontrolled uterine bleeding?

Confusing things even more was a 1940 report in the *American Journal of Psychiatry* on the treatment of five "morbidly oversexed" females with 25 milligrams of testosterone, a dose that was said to be effective, though one of the women "complained bitterly that she was being *de-sexed.*"[25]

As the 1940s moved into the 1950s and testosterone failed at one appointed task after another, marketers beat a forced retreat to promoting it as a treatment for female "frigidity," an epidemic that erupted in the 1950s along with Freudian psychoanalysis, which asserted that the only normal, healthy sex for women was vaginal penetration to the point of orgasm. Women left unsatisfied by this sexual regimen were diagnosed as "frigid," and testosterone was used as a "cure." Both women with unusually active sex lives and those deemed insufficiently active were candidates for medical intervention. But this was before the Pill, before the sexual revolution of the 1960s, and long before the marketing juggernaut that accompanied Viagra. Many doctors and their female patients were uncomfortable on this new terrain, and testosterone sales went nowhere.

As for "male sexual dysfunction," many doctors remained unconvinced that stimulating the sexual appetites of older men was a medical concern. To the contrary, they openly voiced their doubts about the wisdom of helping men who were considered too old to be adequate fathers sire children.

The one thing testosterone did, without question, was produce obvious changes in the human body: muscle growth, facial hair, and lowered voices. This should have come as no surprise, since testosterone had been chemically isolated by correlating its administration to changes in the sizes of rooster combs immediately obvious to the naked eye. Doctors and women alike, however, viewed these visible side effects as worse than whatever benefit the chemical might offer.[26]

Testosterone, the "most secret quintessence of life," fountain of youth, and pharmaceutical gold mine, was a miracle drug without a disease.

3

The "Female Sex Hormone," the Goddess of Fortune

The basic chemical structure common to all the estrogens was elucidated in the early 1920s, much earlier than testosterone. The chief chemist at Organon, the major Dutch corporation in the sex hormone race, dubbed it "the goddess of fortune." But then came the discovery that there were two chemical estrogens produced by the endocrine system, then three. In fact, once chemists started looking for it in earnest, the "female sex hormone" seemed to be everywhere. Already in 1929 one researcher commented that the "female principle which we call the female sex hormone is widely distributed through the vegetable and animal kingdom," including in yeast, the buds of willows, sugar beets, rice, ovaries and placenta, male body fluids including blood, urine, and bile, and even testes.[1]

Drug companies went to work trying out various formulas distilled from urine or extracted from ovaries in search of something marketable. Amniotin, sold by the US firm E. R. Squibb & Sons, was derived from the fetal fluids of cattle.[2] Organon countered with Ovarnon, which they immediately began to sell without any clear idea of what to use it for, and after a "safety trial" with just five participants (three men and two women), one of whom got sick. ("Clinical trials" as we think of them today were yet to be invented.) When clinical use showed no results, Organon increased the dosage, changed the brand name, and tried again.[3]

When Organon first began selling the new drug in 1927, it came recommended for menstrual disorders of limited kinds. This was quickly expanded to menstrual disorders of all kinds, then menopause, then schizophrenia and melancholia, then skin and joint diseases, then epilepsy, hair loss, eye disorders, diabetes, hemophilia, and chilblains. This expansion occurred over just two years, and resulted not from any new knowledge about the effects of the drug but because Organon and its competitors were finding estrogen products hard to sell. The drugs were expensive, since vast amounts of animal fluids or body parts had to be collected to distill even tiny amounts of the preparations, yet they didn't seem to do much (other than cornify the wall of a mouse vagina).

Unlike testosterone, which could be cheaply synthesized in the lab, chemists were stymied in their efforts to create synthetic equivalents of biological estrogens. Then, to everyone's surprise, it was discovered that there were synthetic substances—not produced by any living organism but created in the lab—that were *not* chemically similar to biological estrogens but could cornify the lining of mouse vaginas far more potently than anything produced by living bodies. These chemicals seemed to bond to estrogen receptors just like the estrogens produced by glands, but remained in the bloodstream longer, making them *more estrogenic than estrogens.*

DES and Premarin

The first such synthetic estrogen used on women was bisphenol A (BPA), a chemical that had been kicking around since 1891. BPA's moment at the top of the synthetic estrogen heap was quickly ended by diethylstilbestrol (DES), a newer chemical created in 1938, which was three times as estrogenic as the strongest biological estrogen, as measured by the mouse vagina assay. (BPA went back on the shelf but not for long. It will spectacularly resurface decades down the road in a very different context.)

DES was the creation of Charles Dobbs, a British researcher who was in a tight race for a synthetic estrogen patent with his German counterpart. Dobbs was convinced that Hitler's regime was on the verge of controlling the patent on synthetic estrogen, a cutting-edge technology that seemed to portend nearly magical powers. So Dobbs made an extraordinary move: instead of patenting his formula, he published it. In fact, he rushed it into print. Within months, chemists and drug companies in many countries were working on new "estrogen" products with his formula.[4]

The "goddess of fortune" was revealed to be distilled not from ovaries but from coal tar. DES did not even have a steroid chemical structure like all biologically produced "sex hormones," and as a result it could be manufactured at a fraction of previous cost. DES, then, was not protected by patent, cheap to produce, and could be made in unlimited quantities. Bingo! The torrent of activity unleashed by DES was unlike anything previously seen in medicine. As the feminist historian Barbara Seaman puts it: "Drug manufacturers dreamed about new hormone product lines. They thought menopause. They thought menstruation. They thought beautiful skin, thicker hair, more passionate sex. They thought of curing infertility, preventing miscarriages, and drying up breast milk in mothers who preferred to bottle-feed. Some of the more daring were also thinking birth control."[5] Within months, several pharmaceutical corporations began giving DES away to doctors in large quantities on the condition that they prescribe it for all kinds of ailments and report back what worked.

The most vocal opponent of all this was the chemical's creator, Charles Dodd, who insisted, "We should always be humbled when we think of what we do not know about the female reproductive cycle. . . . We still have to proceed with caution on any long-term hormonal treatment of the human female."[6]

Most troubling were lab results suggesting a link between DES and cancer. In fact, Dodd came up with DES while studying the close chemical similarity between a certain class of carcinogens and one of the biological estrogens secreted by ovaries. Dodd and his research team threw themselves into a series of studies that they again rushed into publication, linking DES with cancer, problems of sexual development, and more.[7]

The drug companies were undeterred, and by 1939 several had applied to the newly strengthened Food and Drug Administration (FDA) for approval of DES (sold under the name stilboestrol) as a treatment for menopause. The ensuing debate became the new agency's first major controversy, which soon escalated into a full-scale political brawl, with multiple drug companies lined up in favor of DES, and many scientists, doctors, and the American Medical Association against. New and troubling studies piled up. Three showed that the offspring of female rats given DES during pregnancy had deformed genitalia and reproductive organs. In 1941 came the first report linking DES with cervical cancer.[8]

The impasse was broken on the pages of *Reader's Digest,* at the time a wildly popular magazine with a circulation of 9 million. A journalist named Helen Haberman announced that "Help for Women over Forty" was on the way, to relieve them of "the most distressing of natural body processes, . . . a dreaded crisis of discomfort and depression."[9] Haberman pointedly noted that the only thing standing in the way between these wretched women and the "sensational" new drug was the FDA. Letters from women demanding access to DES flooded into the FDA and even to President Roosevelt himself at the White House.[10] The FDA approved DES shortly thereafter, albeit only with a doctor's written consent, making the synthetic estrogen one of the first prescription drugs.

Almost immediately, DES encountered serious competition when Ayerst Laboratories announced a product made from the processed urine of pregnant horses. Stallions, if you remember, have more estrogen in their urine than mares, but stallions turned out to be highly uncooperative about having their urine collected, so Ayerst turned to pregnant mares as the next best thing. Harvesting enough raw material for industrial-scale production of Premarin required maintaining vast herds of mares kept in a constant state of pregnancy, but this was hormone gold they would be harvesting, so the effort was sure to pay off. Named Premarin (for PREgnant MARe urINe), the product could cornify the wall of a mouse vagina nearly as potently as DES but without the noxious side effects. Premarin immediately displaced DES as the drug of choice for menopause.

Estrogen from ovaries is to Premarin and DES what an ear of corn is to high fructose corn syrup and saccharin. Corn contains a sugar called glucose, which triggers a response in our bodies we call "sweet." Corn and humans evolved together through vast expanses of time, so we have a pretty good idea how our bodies react to eating corn. Saccharin is a synthetic chemical that triggers a "sweet" response in bodies similar to our response to corn, but the response is far stronger. Since it is synthetic, we don't have to grow it; chemical plants can just churn it out. But since humans (and other organisms) have not evolved eating it, we know very little about what *else* it might trigger in our bodies. High fructose corn syrup is made from corn from a plant, but that corn is industrially processed to concentrate its sugar to a much higher density, and in the process some glucose chemically converts to fructose. Just as the makers of high fructose corn syrup argue that it is safer than artificial sweeteners because it is "natural," Ayerst argued that Premarin was safer than DES, and the relative mildness of its immediate side effects reinforced this perception.

Selling Menopause as a Disease

The FDA approved Premarin for treatment of menopause, but many doctors and women did not view menopause as a disease that required treatment in the first place. Medical advice books of the previous era suggested that the menopausal woman "may look forward to a long and placid period of rest, blessed with health, honored and loved with a purer flame than any which she inspired in the bloom of youth." So before Ayerst could sell the drug, they had to sell the disease. Ad copy played on the idea that a menopausal woman was not "complete" and was "condemned to witness the death of her own womanhood." Doctors were advised to "Keep her on Premarin." One ad showed a man glaring at his deranged wife while comforting his daughter who is on the verge of tears. The ad copy stated: "Almost any tranquilizer might calm her down . . . but at her age estrogen might be what she really needs" for "an improved sense of well-being."[11]

The ads were complemented by the efforts of evangelist doctors. As Robert Battey had done for "normal ovariotomies," so William H. Masters did for Premarin.[12] Masters conducted his research on patients in the St. Louis city infirmary for the indigent, and began publishing after administering hormones to just fifteen elderly female residents over three years. Soon he was administering estrogen to over a hundred women who were vaginal-smeared, biopsied, weighed, measured, photographed, and questioned for years on end. Women with malignant tumors were kept on estrogen nevertheless. At a conference in 1955, Masters himself acknowledged that these women "were, in essence, experimental laboratory animals."

Of his original fifteen women, six died, two showed "no improvement" and were dropped from the cohort, one refused to continue, and three "improved" and, over Masters's objections, were subsequently taken home by their families and thus received no more estrogen treatments. Only three continued with the treatment and showed "improvement," but the measures of "improvement" were as strange as everything else. A big deal was made of mentally ill women who had previously refused to get out of bed becoming ambulatory. The women were given the Thematic Apperception Test, which asked them to make up stories about pictures, and researchers concluded "the experimental group told better stories," and that "if the gains here reported are substantiated in other groups and can be maintained over longer periods of time, it is believed that an avenue of treatment possessing definite psychological benefits for older females in our culture will have been demonstrated." In a separate thirteen-month study, two of the patients died, but there were no deaths among the controls. One died "without prior warning" of a heart attack. As we will see, increased risk for heart attack would later emerge as an extremely contentious issue for estrogen treatment. In spite of mortality rates of 18 percent and 40 percent in the two studies, Masters concluded that the treatment "achieves its effect by what seems to be an arrest, and possibly a partial reversal, of the aging process."

Masters traveled the country issuing a clarion call for keeping postmenopausal women on estrogen for the remainder of their lives to prevent them from falling into what he called "the third sex" or "the neutral gender." Soon he moved beyond even this, calling for " 'puberty to grave' sex steroid support." He extended his vision of lifetime hormone therapy to men as well, arguing that his principles of hormone replacement should be applied to all people without regard to "previous sex." Admittedly, he had not studied hormone therapy in men, but he explained that this was because "females as a sex constitute more of a public health problem than the males due to their greater expected longevity," and because females "are, as a rule, generally more amenable to therapy, repeated biopsies, and examinations than are the males." He added that women lost their gender earlier than men and thus were a larger burden on society: "There are obviously many women who have joined the 'neuter gender' age group before their fiftieth birthday. Equally obviously, there are a significant number of males who could not be considered candidates for the third sex even after their seventieth birthday." An appeal to a sort of medical patriotism became part of his schtick: if everyone in the United States maintained a steady state of estrogen and testosterone in their blood from puberty to death, "a major contribution will have been made, not only to the treated individuals but to the economy and potential manpower supply of our country."

After a decade as the St. Paul of estrogen, Masters moved on to become half of Masters and Johnson, the sexology gurus of the 1970s. He studied "human sexual response" by observing more than ten thousand orgasms between arbitrarily paired research subjects in his lab, and claimed a success rate of 70 percent in his pioneering "conversion therapy" of homosexuals into heterosexuals. That research continues to inform such endeavors today, even though after his death his partner, Virginia Johnson, admitted that Masters had most likely fabricated his homosexual conversion research.[13]

When Masters transitioned from estrogen to orgasms, Dr. Robert Wilson picked up the torch for estrogen and carried it out of medical journals and into the public square with his blockbuster best seller, *Feminine Forever.*[14] Wilson described the postmenopausal woman as part victim and part monster. "The tragedy of menopause often destroys her character along with her health," leaving her a "dull-minded but sharp tongued caricature of her former self" who may "subside into a stupor of indifference."[15] Ayerst actually paid Wilson to write the book, then followed it up with a "Forever Feminine" ad campaign. The next year saw yet another best seller, *Everything You Always Wanted to Know about Sex but Were Afraid to Ask,* by Dr. David Reuben, who described the postmenopausal woman as "not really a man but no longer a functional woman," living "in the world of intersex."[16] By this point Ayerst Laboratories was spending a million dollars a year to advertise Premarin, which had become one of the best-selling prescription medications in the United States.

DES for Mothers, Tall Girls, and Livestock

The sellers of DES did not go quietly into the night after Premarin cornered the menopause market. And there were a lot of them: 250 drug companies eventually manufactured and marketed DES under 325 different names. When Premarin pushed them out of menopause, they switched gears and began promoting DES as a way to reduce the rate of miscarriage and other pregnancy complications. By 1957, advertisements in medical journals recommended DES for *all* pregnancies, not just to prevent miscarriage but to produce "bigger and stronger" babies, or even to "make a normal pregnancy more normal."[17] Once again, the practice was aggressively championed by an evangelizing doctor, in this case Karl John Karnaky in Houston. Charles Dodd, the creator of DES, angrily sent Karnaky a study showing that DES *caused* miscarriages in rabbits and rats, but Karnaky was having none of it. By his own estimate, Karnaky eventually gave DES to 150,000 pregnant women. Administering DES to pregnant women became so common that many hospitals didn't even keep records of the practice, and women were often not told what they were taking. As a result, no one knows how many pregnant women were given DES, but estimates run as high as 2 million.[18]

DES manufacturers probed new markets as well, such as using DES to treat "the problem of excessive height in otherwise normal girls." This effort began with research into using estrogens to treat acromegaly, a potentially life-threatening disease resulting from excess growth hormone production by the anterior pituitary gland. But almost immediately the effort expanded to include adolescent girls with a predicted height just four inches above average. By 1977, a survey of American pediatric endocrinologists found that half of them had treated tall girls with estrogen therapy.[19] A large medical literature accumulated, which dutifully noted adverse side effects of giving estrogen to tall girls, ranging from nausea and headaches all the way to ovarian cysts, hypertension, and blood clots.

DES was also being used to suppress milk production after childbirth, and to treat acne, prostate cancer, and gonorrhea in children. But by this time the profits made from administering DES to humans were dwarfed by the profits from administering it to animals. In 1947 the US Department of Agriculture approved the use of DES in poultry. A pellet of DES implanted in the neck of a chicken or rooster redistributed body fat (just as it did in people), in a manner the poultry industry thought profitable. In 1954, DES was approved for cattle and sheep as well. By 1979 more than 30 million head of cattle (80–95% of US cattle) were being treated with DES, and synthetic estrogen was finally living up to its advance billing as "the goddess of fortune."[20]

Meat, however, is culturally associated with manliness, and all this estrogen in meat made consumers nervous. Drug companies sought to allay these fears by feeding journalists lines like "The housewife need not fear that if her husband eats a stilbestrol chicken he will give up golf and hunting and start knitting sweaters." Workers in chemical and meat-packing plants, farms, and restaurants began experiencing health problems from DES exposure. When one chemical manufacturer wrote to the FDA for advice on how to minimize DES health risks for its production workers, the FDA replied that "exposure to the substances may cause marked disturbances of the menstrual function in women and have a devirilizing effect in men. For this reason it might be feasible for you to consider the employment of old rather than young men."[21]

The Pill

In 1960, the FDA approved the first oral contraceptive. Popularly known as the Pill, it was the culmination of the life work of Margaret Sanger, a radical nurse whose mother had eighteen pregnancies in twenty-two years and died at the age of fifty. Sanger went on a lifelong mission to make each woman "the absolute mistress of her own body." She published *The Woman Rebel* newsletter, opened the nation's first "birth control" clinic (a term she coined), and founded Planned Parenthood. After investigating every kind of contraception, she concluded that the optimal contraceptive would have to be simple to use, inexpensive, and controlled by women. She set her sights on a pill because it could be taken at a time and place of a woman's choosing, away from the sex act and the eyes of men. She followed developments in endocrinology in the 1950s, and enlisted the financial support of a feminist philanthropist to fund the research of a maverick Catholic endocrinologist in a crash program that resulted in the Pill, a mix of synthetic estrogen and progesterone (the "pro-gestational" hormone).[22] This is how it works:

> Briefly, at the start of the reproductive cycle, the pituitary gland at the base of the brain secretes follicle-stimulating hormone (FSH), which stimulates the follicles of the ovary to mature. These ovarian follicles secrete the hormone estrogen, which then stimulates the lining of the uterus to thicken and to become enriched with blood vessels. The pituitary responds to the increasing level of estrogen in the blood by decreasing the secretion of FSH and then secreting luteinizing hormone

(LH), which induces a follicle to rupture and release an egg (ovulation). The ruptured follicle, now called the corpus luteum, secretes the hormone progesterone, which maintains the thickened uterine lining within which a fertilized egg could implant. So long as the corpus luteum is secreting progesterone, the pituitary will not secrete FSH, so other eggs are prevented from maturing. After its release from the ovary, the egg travels through the Fallopian tubes on its way to the uterus. If the egg is fertilized by a sperm, it will implant in the wall the uterus. The fertilized egg then secretes a hormone called chorionic gonadotropin, which maintains the corpus luteum and its secretion of progesterone until the placenta forms and takes over progesterone production. If no egg implants, the corpus luteum breaks down. As the amount of progesterone in the blood decreases, the uterine lining breaks down (menstruation) and the pituitary increases the secretion of FSH to begin another cycle. The pill works primarily by inhibiting ovulation. Synthetic estrogen and progesterone elevate the hormone levels in the blood, preventing the pituitary gland from releasing FSH, so no egg is stimulated to develop within the ovary. The synthetic progesterone component increases the thickness of cervical mucus, incapacitates sperm, slows the movement of the egg, and prevents complete development of the uterine lining. All of these effects provide important contraceptive backups in case hormone levels are not high enough to inhibit ovulation.[23]

Well, not *so* briefly, but the description provides a window on the complexity of the endocrine system. The Pill contains two synthetic hormones that intervene in an enormously complex chain of multiple feedbacks involving five different hormones secreted by three organs and an egg, all tied to the brain. But one thing was certain about the Pill: it worked. Finally the "goddess of fortune" had given birth to a reliable product that had a measurable effect everyone agreed on. The Pill prevented pregnancy. As to what *else* it did, well . . .

The age of marriage rose. The size of families fell. The number of women in higher education and the professions rose. The playwright Clare Boothe Luce declared, "With the Pill, modern woman is at last free, as a man is free, to dispose of her own body, to earn her living, to pursue the improvement of her mind, to try a successful career."[24] And then came the whole "sexual revolution" of the sixties and seventies. The Pill may not have *caused* the sexual revolution, but it would be difficult to imagine the sexual revolution without it.[25]

By 1968, seven different brands of the Pill were racking up $150 million in sales, while the number of estrogen prescriptions written for menopause soared from 15.5 million in 1966 to 28 million in 1975. New prescriptions of Premarin alone hit 5 million in 1974, nearly a million of which were for first-time users.[26] Many women planned to take the synthetic estrogen in the Pill every day of their adult lives (stopping only if a pregnancy was desired), until switching to the processed horse estrogen in Premarin from menopause until death. And throughout it all they could make their "forever feminine" bodies more feminine still with a vast array of estrogen-based cosmetic creams, lotions, and oils. Chemical manufacturers had a particular incentive to develop these products, since cosmetics could be sold without a doctor's prescription and marketed directly to the public in the mainstream media. William H. Masters's "'puberty to grave' sex steroid support," a fringe idea just twenty years before, had become a fact of life.

4

The Estrogen Mess

The era of the Pill also saw the emergence of the "second wave" of feminism in the United States. Many women first encountered the new feminism in women-only discussion groups with like-minded peers. Where to begin the new feminist revolution? Many discussion groups agreed that, as Tish Sommers (founder of the Older Women's League) put it, "Taking control of our own lives and of our bodies is the most basic feminist principle there is."[1] When the women began to discuss bodies and health, they were shocked to discover how much estrogen everyone was taking, on the prescription of male doctors and sold for huge profits by giant corporations run by men. For many, the next step was the startling realization that they were not the only ones feeling negative "side effects" from all that estrogen.

Feminist Reaction

In 1969 Barbara Seaman published *The Doctors' Case against the Pill.* Seaman's transition from columnist for magazines like *Ladies' Home Journal* and *Family Circle* to crusader for women's control of women's bodies was emblematic of the time. Her book was based on interviews with doctors, researchers, and most importantly, women who took the Pill. She reported side effects ranging from heart attacks, strokes, blood clots, and cancer to suicidal depression. What shocked her readers most was not that so many doctors were unaware of these effects, but that those who knew did not share the information with their female patients. Male doctors patronizingly shielded their female patients from the troubling details of their drug regimens.

Seaman's book quickly became a best seller and led to Senate hearings on the Pill the following year. The hearings were disrupted by the members of D.C. Women's Liberation, who objected that none of the many witnesses were women. Today, activist disruptions of Senate hearings are so commonplace as to appear scripted, and the media pays little attention, but in 1970 it was major news. On ABC, the news anchor quoted the testimony of a doctor who recommended that no one take the Pill for more than two years; viewers then saw a film clip in which the same doctor added, "These agents are somewhat like an iceberg. The obvious problems have surfaced in the form of blood clotting disorders. A nagging specter of cancer remains." On CBS News, Walter Cronkite noted, "Almost nine million women in America, and ten million elsewhere, are taking the Pill each day, in the words of one expert, 'as automatically as chickens eating corn.'"[2] Many feminists concluded that, in the words of the activist and writer Gena Corea, "in developing contraceptives, male physicians and researchers have devalued women."[3] Margaret Sanger, who had died only in 1966, must have been rolling over in her grave.

Estrogen, Cancer, and the Women's Health Movement

About the same time, doctors in Boston were stunned to discover seven young women with a form of vaginal cancer (clear-cell adenocarcinoma) so rare that only four occurrences in women under thirty had ever been reported in the medical literature worldwide. From 1969 to 1971 they studied the medical histories of these seven women, along with one additional case they had located, and they discovered that the mothers of seven of the eight had taken DES in the first trimester of pregnancy. They immediately published their finding in *New England Journal of Medicine*. Doctors in New York who read the article searched New York's cancer registry and found five more cases of the same rare cancer in young women whose mothers had taken synthetic estrogen while pregnant, and this was quickly reported in the same journal. Officials in New York soon tracked sixty-two cases of cervical or vaginal adenocarcinoma tied to DES. Researchers called for the creation of a national registry of women who had used DES so that their offspring could be tracked. The *New England Journal of Medicine* published a special editorial on DES and cancer, noting that most of the beef Americans ate came from cows that had been fed DES, and that "there is no way to judging the risk" of eating the meat.[4] DES had even been distributed on some college campuses as a "morning after" contraceptive pill. DES suddenly transitioned from miracle drug to medical emergency.

Even with all of that, the public profile of the DES controversy was minor compared to what occurred four years later when the *New England Journal of Medicine* published two studies showing elevated rates of endometrial cancer (cancer of the uterine lining) among women who took Premarin for menopause. And the risk increased the longer the exposure: women who took estrogen for more than seven years showed a cancer risk fourteen times greater than those who did not. The *Journal's* editors underscored the gravity of the findings by commissioning two editorials on the subject, published along with the research.

Estrogen prescriptions plummeted by half.[5] The DES and Premarin controversies galvanized a national women's health movement that grew to include feminist health centers in many urban areas, the National Women's Health Network, the National Black Women's Health Project, DES Action, and much more.

The connection of estrogen to cancer was challenged by the pharmaceutical industry, and a flurry of research to clarify the matter ensued. Studies piled up, each seeming to contradict the conclusions of the one before, and instead of a clear understanding of the effects of estrogen treatment on the body, what emerged was a rift over epistemological issues as fundamental as whether causality can be established by statistical correlation, what constitutes disease, and ultimately what qualifies as scientific knowledge.

Osteoporosis: Bones to Pick

The estrogen industry retreated, retooled, and came roaring back. Progestin was added to the estrogen used for long-term hormone replacement therapy (HRT) on the theory that this would reduce the risk of cancer. Concurrently, a lavishly financed campaign promoting estrogen therapy for osteoporosis was launched. This was not the result of any new data or research concerning the relationship between estrogen levels and bone loss. The relevant research had been around since 1940.[6] Rather, the old research was brought out of mothballs to support a marketing strategy built on the argument that the increase in cancer risk from estrogen therapy should be balanced against its benefit in decreasing risk of osteoporosis.

Osteoporosis became the disease of the eighties, with a new round of magazine features, advice books, and media interviews on menopause and osteoporosis. In 1982 only 15 percent of the population could identify osteoporosis. Five years later that figure had leaped to 85 percent. Osteoporosis acquired the rhetorical dimensions of a national crisis. The *Journal of Medicine* declared, "Postmenopausal osteoporosis is a major public health problem in the United States today." *Medical World News* measured the "toll in health care dollars" from osteoporosis at "nearly $4 billion a year." Senators close to the pharmaceutical lobby organized hearings, and shortly thereafter the *Federal Register* announced the revised classification of estrogen as "effective for the treatment of postmenopausal osteoporosis."[7]

Given the scale of the alleged osteoporosis calamity, it was inevitable that the conversation would turn from treatment to prevention, and prevention required a way to determine who was at risk. Bone density mass was proposed as the screen, and soon women across the country were having their bone densities measured, often followed by prescriptions for estrogen.

Industry critics responded as best they could. The National Women's Health Network warned, "There is a danger that existing treatment for osteoporosis may be mass marketed and that women will once again be guinea pigs for medical treatments which could prove to be fatal."[8] Researchers found no correlation between bone density measurements and actual bone problems. Soon a debate over whether osteoporosis was a disease or merely an aspect of the female aging process took its place next to the debate over whether menopause was a disease or merely an aspect of the female aging process.

Every middle-aged woman was now expected to analyze the risks and benefits of estrogen treatment and make "the hormone therapy decision," the title of an entire chapter of *Women Coming of Age* by the celebrity actress Jane Fonda.[9] Taking a page from the women's health movement, hospitals and private clinics hosted menopause seminars and discussion groups to help patients weigh their options, but critics charged these were just one more way that for-profit medicine co-opted activism to sell drugs. Those most informed perceived a divide between the "medical model" and "feminist model" of menopause and aging, but in fact it became harder to cast the debate as one between feminism and patriarchy. Women physicians, who had begun to increase in number, prescribed HRT more often than their male counterparts and were more likely than other women to take HRT themselves. On one side, *Ms.* magazine scoffed at the "full-scale launch of the meno-boom, inundating women with 'information' that detailed all the loss, misery, humiliation, and despair suddenly in store for us."[10] On the other, Gail Sheehy, author of a best-selling book advocating HRT, called her critics "women frozen in an outdated era of feminism" who were "more dangerous than the wrong drug."[11]

Many women who had been on HRT prior to 1975 found it difficult to give up their estrogen, especially if they had been using it for many years or tried to quit "cold turkey."[12] Others insisted they were pleased with the benefits they got from estrogen, and worried that their post-menopausal lives would be intolerable without it. But no one could agree on how to measure the benefits of HRT. Studies showed, for example, that women who took estrogen long-term also exercised more and ate better than women who did not take estrogen. Diet and exercise had been the recommended treatment for menopausal symptoms before the era of estrogen.

The migration of the debate from the cloistered world of medicine to the public marketplace, which had begun with the magazine columns and advice books of prior decades, accelerated when the FDA approved "direct-to-consumer" drug advertising in 1985, and relaxed the restrictions on product-specific television ads in 1997. The amount of money spent on what is now called DTC advertising by the drug industry skyrocketed from $12 million in 1989 to $156 million in 1992, $595 million in 1996, and $1.58 billion in 1999, a 130-fold increase in just ten years. In 1998, $37.1 million was spent on DTC advertising for Premarin alone. Book publishing proceeded apace. In one three-year span more than one hundred books were published on the subject of menopause.[13]

By 1988, Premarin had clawed its way up the profit chain to fifth most frequently prescribed drug. Four years later it hit number one and stayed at the top of the charts every year for the rest of the century. HRT prescriptions rose from 36.5 million in 1992 to 58.3 million in 1995, 75.8 million in 1997, and 89.6 million in 1999.[14] The number of mares kept perpetually pregnant so that their urine could be harvested to supply these nearly 100 million prescriptions was estimated at 40,000.[15] (In 2009, Premarin's manufacturer, Wyeth, would be purchased for $68 billion by the pharmaceutical giant Pfizer, largely because of its ownership of Premarin. In response to a growing campaign among animal rights activists in the United States and Canada protesting the treatment of horses in Premarin production, Pfizer would move production to China and double the number of horses.)[16]

As estrogen use rebounded, so did the rhetoric of "the anti-aging lifestyle." *Ladies' Home Journal,* the former employer of Barbara Seaman, declared: "This is the best of all times for women. We have come into our own in an age of scientific breakthrough and medical miracles. But women, not surprisingly, always want more . . . not only longer lives, but health and beauty, too. With science as our handmaiden, we may yet achieve that Eden . . . [as] cosmetic companies compete with pharmaceutical companies to develop more effective products."[17]

The Women's Health Initiative

Studies piled up. By 1991 at least thirty studies had been published on HRT and breast cancer, while upwards of twenty more reported on estrogen use and heart disease.[18] Many of the latter produced conflicting results, but estrogen marketers nevertheless added lower risk of heart disease to their list of estrogen's alleged benefits, which now included alleviating the negative symptoms of menopause, rejuvenating the skin, and reducing the risk of both osteoporosis and heart disease. The big-ticket items on the list of negatives were elevated risk of endometrial and breast cancer. Each and every one of these claims was contested, but the drug companies thought the addition of heart disease on the plus side looked like a clincher.

Feminists countered that no drug had ever been prescribed for heart disease in men without first passing safety trials, so why were doctors prescribing estrogen as a heart disease drug for women without the same? Finally, in 1991, Bernadine Healy, the first woman to run the

National Institutes of Health (NIH), took the bull by the horns and launched the Women's Health Initiative (WHI), a $625 million study to compare the risks and benefits of hormone treatment, low-fat diet, and dietary supplements like calcium and vitamin D. All told, the project encompassed forty clinical centers and seven coordinating centers in twenty-seven states working over fourteen years with 160,000 subjects. There was grumbling about the study being an unconscionable waste of resources spent to "prove" what chemists and doctors already knew, all to placate a small bunch of shrill feminists, but the grumblers hoped the trial would finally lay to rest the whole bugaboo concerning the safety of estrogen.

In 2002 the NIH stunned the medical world by shutting down the arm of the WHI testing Prempro, a member of what was now the "Premarin family" and the top-selling HRT drug. Trial data showed that Prempro increased the risk of breast cancer to the point that it would be unethical to continue giving it to test subjects. Prempro also increased risk for heart disease by 29 percent. Prempro was the estrogen drug to which the pharmaceutical giant Wyeth had added progestin in order to reduce the cancer risk associated with estrogen alone. Estrogen and progestin were also the two components of the Pill.

Millions of women stopped taking estrogen overnight. The stock of Wyeth, Prempro's maker, fell 24 percent. Sales of all estrogen products plummeted. Recommendations for estrogen use were revised. HRT was now advised only when menopausal symptoms are severe, and then for as brief a time as possible.

But that was just the beginning.

In 2003 the NIH announced that subsequent analysis showed that Prempro not merely failed to protect from mild memory loss, as some had claimed, but women taking it were at increased risk for dementia.

In 2004 the other shoe dropped when the estrogen-only arm was shut down because the subjects showed an increased risk of stroke. Long-term estrogen use was revealed to be so dangerous that it was unethical to experiment with it on humans.

Though the administration of hormones was now suspended in both arms of the massive Women's Health Initiative, the NIH continued to track the health of the study participants, and issued regular updates as time went by:

- 2006: Estrogen-only treatment does not increase the risk of breast cancer in postmenopausal women.
- 2007: Estrogen and estrogen-plus-progestin may reduce heart disease in women who start therapy closer to menopause.
- 2009: Estrogen-plus-progestin for more than five years doubles the risk of breast cancer.
- 2011: Women who took estrogen alone had 46 percent fewer heart attacks and a smaller reduction for risk in breast cancer.
- 2013: The WHI's final report concludes, "Menopausal hormone therapy has a complex pattern of risks and benefits. Findings from the intervention and extended postintervention follow-up of the 2 WHI hormone therapy trials do not support use of this therapy for chronic disease prevention, although it is appropriate for symptom management in some women."[19]

At the time of the final report in 2013, the only unambiguous conclusion that could be drawn from the WHI was that older postmenopausal women who begin HRT (the main target market for estrogen drugs for half a century) dramatically increase their risk for heart attack, stroke, breast cancer, and other complications. The finding that estrogen alone reduces heart attacks and breast cancer has little clinical implication, since estrogen alone damages the uterus, so only women without a uterus take estrogen alone. Progestin blunts the harmful effects of estrogen on the uterus, but reverses the reduction of risk for heart attack and breast cancer associated with estrogen alone.

Fifteen years and $625 million after it had begun, the Women's Health Initiative seemed to have cleared up nothing. The debates around estrogen were more unsettled than ever. They were also louder and more acrimonious, involving more drugs, and more claims of benefits and liabilities, nearly all of which remained contested.

DES Redux

We now return to the story of synthetic estrogen, picking up where we left off in the 1970s when DES taken during pregnancy was linked to an extremely rare form of vaginal cancer. In 1980 the FDA banned the use of DES in livestock. The same year, the Supreme Court issued a landmark decision imposing a "rebuttable presumption of market share liability" on all DES manufacturers, proportional to their market share at the time the drug was consumed by the mother of a particular plaintiff.[20] An avalanche of lawsuits ensued that continues today at full force. In 2015, thirty-five years after the Supreme Court ruling, a Google search for "DES" revealed an entire army of law firms eager to represent anyone claiming injury from DES. The last remaining DES manufacturer in the United States stopped production in 1997—not because the substance was banned (it wasn't), but because of all the lawsuits.

The difficulties confronting the ongoing research into the consequences of the DES debacle are formidable. No good records were kept of who received it, and many who did were not informed what it was. Beyond that, no one has any idea how to measure exposure from meat. Since there are long lag times before effects are manifest and many effects do not appear until the second generation (the children of exposed women), there are enormous difficulties tracking subjects. More recent studies are expanding the scope of research to include third-generation subjects (grandchildren of women who took DES).

In 1975 the National Cancer Institute launched the first government-sponsored study of "DES-exposed female offspring." Three years later the US Department of Health, Education, and Welfare convened a National DES Task Force. Since 2003, the federal Center for Disease Control has maintained an extensive operation providing information for DES Mothers, DES Daughters, DES Sons, and more recently, DES Grandchildren. Numerous research groups labor at the mammoth job of continuing to track the offspring, and offspring of offspring, of women given DES. There is a national nonprofit organization, DES Action, as well as local support groups scattered around the country. In 1985 President Ronald Reagan declared a national "DES Awareness Week."

The results of DES studies remain every bit as contested and controversial as the HRT studies that proceeded in parallel over the last thirty years. Data from the National Cancer Institute published in 2011 shows DES daughters at increased risk for infertility, spontaneous abortion, preterm delivery, loss of second-trimester pregnancy, ectopic pregnancy, preeclampsia, stillbirth, early menopause, cervical intraepithelial neoplasia, breast cancer, uterine fibroids, and incompetent cervix.[21]

Consequences for DES sons are even more contentious, and while many studies have suggested links to testicular cancer, infertility, and urogenital abnormalities such as cryptorchidism and hypospadias, federal authorities do not consider these outcomes to be confirmed.

Research concerning possible psychological effects of prenatal DES exposure is even more contested. Studies have suggested links to schizophrenia, anxiety disorders, anorexia, and more. Some research has linked "gender dysphoria" or "transsexual outcomes" to prenatal DES exposure.[22] Much of this research has been compiled by male-to-female transexual doctors, who in 2004 launched a DES Trans support group. The appearance of highly educated transexual doctors claiming their trans identity to be the result of synthetic estrogen poisoning has been a wild curve ball thrown into an already dizzyingly complex playing field.

Endocrine Disrupting Chemicals

Observers of the DES controversy might have thought it impossible to imagine an even higher-decibel food fight over these issues, but in recent years just such a fight has erupted over bisphenol A (BPA). BPA, remember, was the first synthetic estrogen. When DES proved more potent, BPA was put back on the shelf until the 1950s, when it was found to be useful in the manufacture of plastic, epoxy, dental sealants, and the lining of food and beverage containers. Thus the exact same chemical is considered either an estrogen or an industrial additive, depending on who is using it for what purpose. And there are now huge amounts of plastic and food and beverage containers containing BPA dispersed across the surface of the planet. As BPA became ubiquitous throughout industrial society and beyond, evidence accumulated that it was "disrupting" the endocrine systems of those exposed. Since BPA had been the first synthetic chemical deliberately used for its estrogenic effects, this should have come as no surprise, but the early history of BPA had been long forgotten. A review of BPA by the National Institutes of Health, published in 2010, expressed "some concern for effects on the brain, behavior, and prostate gland in fetuses, infants, and children at current human exposures to bisphenol A." The NIH attempted to clarify this ambiguous statement by explaining their scale of "levels of concern about the different effects of chemicals: negligible concern, minimal concern, some concern, concern, and serious concern."[23]

As of 2016, BPA has been banned from certain products—most often baby bottles—in Europe, Canada, Malaysia, and even China (where regulation of toxic chemicals is notoriously lax). In the United States, where an enormous campaign on BPA's behalf has been mobilized by the chemical industry, the FDA banned BPA from baby bottles and children's drinking cups (2012) and infant formula packaging (2013), and there is also a hodgepodge of local and state regulations.

BPA is now considered just one of a large class of substances termed endocrine disrupting chemicals (EDCs). Many industrially produced synthetic chemicals, it turns out, have estrogenic effects in the body. These chemicals are designed to remain stable throughout industrial manufacturing processes, and as a result they remain "persistent" once they have escaped the confines of their initial product and have gone feral in the big wide world. As the output of the global chemical industry grew from near zero at the dawn of the twentieth century to a relentless deluge at century's end, EDCs accumulated in sewage, farm run-off, industrial waste, human and animal waste, and so on. Today these chemicals can be found everywhere on the face of the earth, and there are no humans left who do not have some of these chemicals in their blood, even if they live in the remotest areas far from industrial production. Essentially, the whole earth is now "on estrogen." In fact, we can say that at the most general level, the chemical consequences of industrialization are that the atmosphere is more heat absorptive, sea water more acidic, and living tissue more estrogenic.

If research on estrogens deliberately consumed for medical purposes faces daunting hurdles, research on estrogens inadvertently consumed from environmental exposure confronts even more. Medical research must deal with issues like how to infer causality from correlation, how to precisely track difference in outcome between exposures at different times in an organism's life, how to track subjects over the long delay between exposure and result (spanning second and even third generations), and how to measure behavioral outcomes. EDC research must deal with all of that plus how to measure doses received from environmental sources, and how to pinpoint when exposure occurred, how to construct control groups in a world where no living being outside the lab is unexposed, among many other things.

As if that were not enough, EDC research is perceived as a threat not just to one company making one drug like Premarin, but to the entire chemical industry and indeed the industrial way of life. As a result, the chemical industry has mobilized a network of researchers, think tanks, and media consultants to "debunk" the whole notion of endocrine disrupting chemicals. This network consists of many of the same individuals and institutions mobilized by the tobacco industry to "debunk" the link between cigarette smoking and cancer, and by climate change denialists to "debunk" the idea that the earth is warming due to industrially produced greenhouse gases. EDCs have been linked to cancer, birth defects, cognitive and brain development disorders, deformations of the body including limbs and reproductive organs, declining fertility rates, and more. Each and every one of these effects is highly contested. Depending on who you listen to, EDCs constitute a global crisis as profound as global warming, a minor problem with less than dire consequences, or a figment of a paranoid environmentalist imagination.

5

The Testosterone Comeback

And testosterone? The "most secret quintessence of life," the search for which started the whole endocrine ball rolling? In the 1950s, after failing to find any disease it could treat, testosterone disappeared into—of all places—the East German police state.

East German Sports Doping

During the Cold War, every aspect of life in East Germany was examined by the state for its potential to demonstrate the superiority of communism. The chemical industry of pre–World War II Germany had been on the cutting edge of the race to synthesize estrogen and testosterone, and the communist authorities in East Germany put that infrastructure to work creating superhuman athletes who for a time dominated certain international sports. Suspicions about the extent of East German sports doping simmered for years, as the little country of 17 million raked in Olympic gold medals: nine in 1968, twenty in 1972, and forty in 1976. In 1993 the East German state and its Berlin Wall collapsed. Long-secret files were opened to the public, revealing a state-run sports doping program on a scale few had imagined. The program was actually overseen by the Stasi, the gargantuan secret police force that grew to employ 2.5 percent of the population spying on the rest. The Stasi kept meticulous records of the drugs' impact on performance, and a top-secret committee, which included members of the high-ranking Parteibüro, met to decide which athlete would be given which drug.[1] Children as young as ten were given testosterone without knowing what it was. Refusing the shots or pills was not an option. Estimates of how many people received testosterone without their consent or knowledge run as high as ten thousand.[2] The East German state was creating the "new socialist man" of communist theory in ways hardly imagined by Marx and Engels.

The testosterone used by the Stasi was what is now known as an anabolic-androgenic steroid: anabolic because it builds tissue, and androgenic because it "virilizes" the body, lowering the voice and stimulating facial hair. The drug of choice in East Germany was Oral-Turinabol, which was initially distilled from hog bile and later made synthetically.[3] The relation of the hog-bile and synthetic versions of Oral-Turinabol to the testosterone produced by the human body parallel the relation of Premarin and DES to human estrogens. And the legacy of the Stasi's doping program in present-day Germany parallels the legacy of DES in the United States. Mountains of unsettled lawsuits remain piled up. Researchers attempt to track the health of athletes-turned-victims who suffer from liver tumors, heart disease, testicular and breast cancer, gynecological problems, infertility, high blood pressure, diabetes, chronic pain, nerve damage, kidney problems, depression, undesired hair growth, eating disorders, miscarriages, and pregnancies resulting in children born with deformities like club feet. The Doping Victim Aid Association helps connect victims with services. One difference, however, is that those at the top of the East German doping operation have been criminally tried and convicted. Nothing of the kind has occurred regarding the manufacture and sale of DES in the United States.

Among the high-profile doping victims is Heidi Krieger, the 1986 European women's shot-put champion, who was systematically drugged beginning at age sixteen. By the time she was eighteen, she weighed 220 pounds and had a deep voice and facial hair. By age thirty-three, Krieger's body had become so masculine in appearance that she requested sex reassignment surgery and changed her—now his—name to Andreas. Andreas now takes testosterone to make his irreversibly masculine appearance more convincing. Krieger's 1986 gold medal has been refashioned into a trophy that looks like a steroid molecule, awarded annually to Germans involved in anti-doping efforts.[4]

The Comeback Kid

The same year the Stasi files were opened in Germany, testosterone sales in the United States began a sudden and rapid rise unlike anything in pharmaceutical history, which has continued to accelerate. Amazingly, as of 2015 there had not been a single new study, or new data of any kind, linking testosterone to efficacious treatment of any disease. To the contrary, there was considerable new data highlighting testosterone's *dangers.* Nevertheless, a series of developments in seemingly unrelated fields came together in a highly combustible mix that fueled testosterone's sudden ascent from the depths of the pharmaceutical market to its pinnacle.

Sports doping. Even as East German athletes began telling their stories and seeking restitution in reunified Germany, athletes in the United States were going to great lengths to secure access to the same dope. The pioneers on the frontier of this endeavor were fanatical body builders who worked out at Gold's Gym near Venice Beach in Southern California, the same gym that won minor notoriety in *Pumping Iron,* the 1979 documentary about Arnold Schwarzenegger. Gold's hosted a covert drug market supplied by drug company sales reps who made money on the side selling samples to weight lifters. In 1982, two gym regulars typed up an eighteen-page how-to manual for black-market testosterone. "We're going to tell you how to keep your doctor happy with your health while you are on steroids," they began, before offering reviews and prices for twenty-nine testosterone-based drugs circulating in the sports underground. Useful tidbits included, "Anavar doesn't make you all that big, it makes you very strong." They printed a few copies in a friend's garage, slapped on a cover that announced *The Underground Steroid Handbook,* placed a tiny ad for their pamphlet in *Muscle Builder & Power* magazine, rented a PO box, and waited. Three months later they had sold eighty thousand copies and pocketed $500,000.[5]

Soon entrepreneurial bodybuilders from the gym were forming illicit partnerships with Mexican black-marketeers to produce an array of testosterone knockoffs that pervaded the world of elite sports, from long-distance runners to NFL linemen to "professional wrestling" superheroes.[6] These drugs then trickled down to amateurs, until by the end of the millennium 2.5 percent of eighth-grade boys had tried "T."[7] The eighteen-page *Handbook* had been replaced by Steroid.com, a website listing 120 "testosterone derivatives," complete with reviews, price lists, and suggested sources in the white, gray, and black markets. The reviews claimed very precise effects: one formulation would make a sprinter faster off the blocks, while another increased stamina for marathons. Doping scandals rocked baseball, football, long-distance cycling, and many Olympic events.

AIDS. Testosterone finally acquired a medicinal use when it proved effective in arresting or even reversing AIDS Wasting Syndrome, an extreme loss of lean body mass common in patients with advanced AIDS. Wasting Syndrome took such a toll on AIDS patients during the worst years of the epidemic that many doctors with large AIDS practices in big urban centers began prescribing testosterone prophylactically to *all* their AIDS patients. HIV-negative gay men began feeling puny working out at the gym next to their HIV-positive friends and lovers, a problem that was easy to remedy given the amount of legally prescribed testosterone circulating through the gay male community. Soon the superhuman physiques of the Gold's Gym at Venice Beach were on full display at gay gyms in Manhattan and San Francisco, as well as in the Internet porn that increasingly set the bar for who qualified as "hot" in the gay male world.

The privatization of medicine. The increasing polarization of wealth combined with the morass of health insurance restrictions and HMO reimbursement schemes to fuel an exodus of doctors out of HMOs and into private, for-profit clinics specializing in high-profit fields like fertility and geriatrics. In 1993 the American Academy of Anti-Aging Medicine was founded with twelve members. By 2012 membership had skyrocketed to 24,000 doctors gathered under the slogan "Aging is NOT inevitable—Together, we can END AGING in our own lifespan."[8] Much of the action is concentrated in male "rejuvenation" clinics springing up across the country, often organized in corporate chains like Ageless Men's Health. In 2012 the chain had fifteen clinics. By 2016 the number was thirty-three. One forty-three-year-old patient who acknowledged that he had no obvious symptoms of low testosterone levels told a reporter, "Am I making a deal with the devil? A little bit, but I have to think about my quality of life. It is like I'm in my 20s again."[9]

Viagra, Addyi, and the medicalization of sex. Beginning with the epidemic of female "frigidity" that followed the ascent of Freudian psychoanalysis in the mid-twentieth century, and continuing through the media blitz accompanying the introduction of Viagra in 1998, doctors gradually shed their discomfort with sexual stimulants. A new diagnosis came into prominence: Inhibited Sexual Desire. By 1990 this had been rechristened as the more clinically authoritative Hypoactive Sexual Desire Disorder (HSDD), which was in turn placed under the umbrella of "sexual dysfunction," clinically defined as "engaging in sexual activities (including masturbation) or having sexual thoughts, fantasies, or urges less than twice a month."[10] At the dawn of the twentieth century, masturbation was a disease. At the century's close, *not* masturbating was a disease.

In 2015 the FDA approved Addyi, or flibanserin, the "female Viagra," to treat HSDD in premenopausal women, even though the fifth edition of the *Diagnostic and Statistical Manual of Mental Disorders* had replaced HSDD with Male Hypoactive Sexual Desire Disorder and Female Sexual Interest/Arousal Disorder. So the new drug was approved to treat a diagnosis that no longer existed. Flibanserin was developed as an antidepressant but was repurposed by its original maker; when it failed to win FDA approval in 2010 the rights were sold to Sprout Pharmaceuticals. Sprout ran new trials and hired a well-known feminist lobbyist to promote the drug in Washington. These trials showed that women receiving flibanserin increased the number of their "satisfying sexual events" from 2.8 to 4.5 a month. The placebo group reported an increase from 2.7 to 3.7 times a month. In other words, flibanserin gave women eight-tenths of a "satisfying sexual event" a month. The main argument put forward in favor of flibanserin's approval seemed to be that since men have Viagra, it would be sexist for the FDA to not approve flibanserin.[11]

HRT and the medicalization of life. In the last decades of the twentieth century, prescription drug sales snowballed into an unprecedented avalanche of chemicals. By 2010 in the United States, one in four children under twelve, nearly one in three teenagers, and nine in ten people over sixty were on at least one prescription drug, and more than a third of the over-sixty group were taking five drugs or more. Americans spent more than $307 billion on prescription drugs in 2010, more than double the total (in constant dollars) less than a decade before, which was already a vast increase from a decade before that.[12] Much of the growth in pharmaceutical sales came from drugs that modified behavior, ranging from antidepressants to a whole collection of drugs for a relatively recent disease called Attention Deficit Hyperactivity Disorder. Marketing the drugs involved not just selling chemicals, but also selling *the idea that behavior was a medical problem treatable with chemicals.*

Media and advertising. In 2000, the conservative gay political columnist Andrew Sullivan recounted his experience with the testosterone his doctor prescribed for AIDS Wasting Syndrome in a lengthy cover story for the *New York Times Magazine,* adding his name to the nearly century-old tradition of hormone-touting blockbuster authors:

> I weighed around 165 pounds. I now weigh 185 pounds. My collar size went from a 15 to a 17 1/2 in a few months; my chest went from 40 to 44. My appetite in every sense of that word expanded beyond measure. Going from napping two hours a day, I now rarely sleep in the daytime and have enough energy for daily workouts and a hefty work schedule. I can squat more than 400 pounds. Depression, once a regular feature of my life, is now a distant memory. . . . I can actually feel [testosterone's] power on almost a daily basis. . . . It is less edgy than a double espresso, but just as powerful. . . . In a word, I feel braced. For what? It scarcely seems to matter. . . . You realize more acutely than before that lust is a chemical.[13]

Sullivan recounted that a forty-year-old executive who took testosterone for bodybuilding purposes told him, "I walk into a business meeting now and I just exude self-confidence. I know there are lots of other reasons for this, but my company has just exploded since my treatment. I'm on a roll. I feel capable of almost anything."

Drug companies couldn't buy publicity like that for any price, but they spent boatloads of money on the kinds of publicity they *could* buy. Their range of options dramatically expanded in 1997 when the FDA made it easier for them to hawk their wares directly to consumers via broadcast media, as part of what is known as DTC marketing. The impact of this decision on the world of prescription drugs was akin to the impact of the 2010 "Citizens United" Supreme Court decision on the electoral politics. The year after the FDA ruling, pharmaceutical companies poured $1.3 billion into DTC advertising, then spent that plus a half billion more in 1999. By 2006 the yearly total was $5.5 billion.[14]

Most of this money was pumped into a handful of chemicals that drug companies thought would be an easy sell to people who spend a lot of time watching TV. Testosterone was high on the list. Abbot spent $20.8 million on testosterone advertising in 2011 alone, much of it on television ads directing viewers to the "Is It Low T?" website, which featured a "Low T Quiz" that would return a "low T" diagnosis to pretty much anyone who answered the questions honestly.[15] A multitude of other sites with more obscured links to major corporations offer diagnostic advice like "If guys don't get a night or waking erection almost every day, then your testosterone level is too low—even if you are in your seventies!"[16] There is even a new literature, both medical and popular, on the national scourge of osteoporosis among American men with "low T." Male osteoporosis now comes flanked by an army of websites offering advice, online diagnosis, and of course, testosterone.[17]

Google searches for "Is It Low T?" return page after page of YouTube videos, corporate fronts, "medical" webzines and more, all featuring wise men in white coats, stethoscopes dangling from their necks like medical bling, pontificating on the national epidemic of low testosterone, and offering sympathetic advice for its victims, along with links to clinics and spas that would sell you the goods.[18] Or you could just skip all that and order the "T" online with a credit card for delivery through the mail. There was a new acronym for testosterone replacement therapy, TRT, coined to parallel HRT for women. Many sites claim that the "male climacteric" kicks in at *thirty years of age,* more than doubling the potential market for testosterone replacement.[19] This would have shocked even William H. Masters, who insisted, "Obviously, there are a significant number of males who could not be considered candidates for the third sex even after their seventieth birthday. It is fair to generalize that the female will be a third-sex candidate roughly fifteen years ahead of the male."[20]

The "Low T" onslaught has led to an increasingly shrill debate among medical professionals that closely mirrors the decades of debate about HRT for women, and the issues at the center of both debates are the same. Is testosterone deficiency is a disease? What would constitute its diagnosis? How could efficacy of treatment be measured? How to balance risks and benefits?

In 2010, the *New England Journal of Medicine* ran reports of two new testosterone studies, along with an editorial. One study concluded that valid diagnostic criteria for "late-onset hypogonadism" (testosterone deficiency) would include testosterone blood levels below a certain number plus "poor morning erection, low sexual desire, and erectile dysfunction," but the accompanying editorial pointed out that many men with testosterone levels that met this criteria reported no sexual problems, while more than 25 percent of men with normal testosterone levels did report the sexual symptoms, and that was before you even got to the problem of how to define "poor morning erection" or "low sexual desire." The other article reported on a study of testosterone replacement therapy in elderly men. While the men receiving testosterone showed marked improvements in leg-press and chest-press strength and in stair climbing while carrying a load, they also had higher rates of "cardiac, respiratory, and dermatologic events." The cardiac side effects were so serious that the trial was deemed unethical and suspended.[21]

Outside of the confines of elite medical research, the multiplying Internet sites yammering about "low T" were countered by handful of sites hosted by government agencies or public universities that seemed almost quaint by comparison. One such site hosted at the University of California at Berkeley valiantly attempt to make its case:

- No one knows what the optimal levels [of testosterone] are.
- Estimates of how many older men have low levels for their age vary widely—from 5% to 35%.
- Low testosterone, however it's defined, is not a problem unless it is accompanied by undesirable symptoms.
- Most men who have sexual symptoms have what's considered normal levels of testosterone. Moreover, most men with low testosterone levels suffer few, if any, related problems.
- Low testosterone is also often associated with conditions such as diabetes, bone loss, obesity, and high blood pressure. But it's not certain whether low testosterone is a cause or an effect of these conditions, or whether supplemental testosterone can ameliorate them.
- Testosterone therapy has been linked to an increased risk of prostate cancer and heart disease, along with liver damage, sleep apnea, breast growth, and prostate enlargement.[22]

There have not been any large long-term clinical trials on testosterone therapy, along the lines of the Women's Health Initiative study on menopausal hormone therapy. That study upended many hopes and beliefs when it found that the hormones had few benefits and actually posed serious risks.

The fact that the "male sex hormone" caused breast growth in men was perhaps the final irony, as if one were needed.

None of this was having much effect on testosterone sales. New uses of the drug were popping up everywhere. Scandals and investigations of testosterone use among police hit one city after another across the nation.[23] A middle-aged female business executive reported that she had gone "from being a driven and outgoing business executive to a paranoid wife" after her start-up software company went bust, but with testosterone treatment her confidence soared and she "aggressively" rebuilt her company. A British gynecologist reported prescribing testosterone implants for female politicians "who want to compete better with their male colleagues in committee meetings and parliamentary debates."[24]

Prescription sales of testosterone increased 500 percent over ten years beginning in 1993, then grew another 115 percent in just five years beginning in 2005. In 2009 annual sales hit nearly $1 billion, then leapfrogged again to $1.6 billion in 2011.[25] "T" was the hottest ticket in the drug business. Giant corporations scrambled to get a piece of the action. One corporate giant, Abbott Laboratories, paid $6.6 billion to acquire the maker of AndroGel. By that time the FDA had also approved Endo Pharmaceuticals' Fortesta, Eli Lilly's Axiron, Actavis's Androderm, and Auxilium's Testim, the last of which was already making $633 million.[26] In 2012, Abbott pumped $80 million into direct-to-consumer advertising for AndroGel, as sales of testosterone gels hit a yearly total of $2 billion. Market analysts were predicting that sales would triple to $5 billion by 2017.[27]

After fifty years languishing on the ropes and nearly falling out of the ring, the "male sex hormone" had come back swinging, suddenly looking like the heavyweight champ it was predicted to be when it first appeared on the scene nearly a century before.

6

"Sex Hormones" Redux —
Not Yours, Your Mother's

While the use of "sex hormones" among the general population grew by leaps and bounds, the debate about their role in shaping both sexual desire and gender identity, or one's sense of being male or female, man or woman, continued unabated.

By the middle of the twentieth century, the testicles of homosexual men had been excised, assayed, sliced, crushed, examined for "F-cell" lesions, and swapped for testicles from both "complete men" and males of other species. But no matter how hard researchers looked, no difference between homosexual testicles and "normal" testicles could be found. Researches then turned their gaze from the testicles to bodily fluids: if the source of the pathology in the testicles remained elusive, perhaps its effects could be measured in the mix of hormones circulating in homosexual blood or expelled in homosexual piss. Blood and urine were examined in microscopic detail but yielded nothing. Homosexual men were just as blue-blooded as everyone else, and they pissed the same yellow fluid that other men pissed. Treatment of male homosexuality remained just as stymied. After testosterone was synthesized, testicle transplants were traded in for testosterone injections, but mainlining the stuff proved no more effective at "curing" male homosexuality than transplanting the organs that secreted it.

In the 1950s the Prague Institute for Sexual Science ran the most comprehensive study ever done measuring physical differences between

94

homosexual and heterosexual men. Everything from the diameter of the areola to longitudinal axis of the testicles was precisely measured. The results showed homosexual male bodies to be exactly the same as heterosexual male bodies except for one detail: homosexuals had larger penises. This was such a black eye for the idea that male homosexuals were "feminized" men, and for manhood in general, that no further such measurements have been made.[1] Thus, as it stands today and has stood for over half a century, the scientific record shows that the only visible difference between gay men and straight is that the former are better endowed.

So much for Magnus Hirschfeld's declaration fifty years before that "of the fifteen hundred homosexuals I have seen, each was physically and mentally distinct from a complete male."

There appears to be not a single study anywhere probing the ovaries, diameter of the areola, or size of the clitoris for the source of homosexuality in women. Apparently, lesbians simply failed to capture the imaginations of the men doing the measuring.

But far from receding in the face of these failures, the search for the hormonal source of homosexuality leaped into a scale of operations that would have stunned old Hirschfeld himself. Just as the hunt for the source of homosexuality in the testicles and blood ground to a disappointing halt, the hunt for the source of homosexuality in the womb began. Hormones could still be the cause of homosexuality, but perhaps the hormones in question were not those in the blood and urine of homosexuals, nor even in their glands that secrete them, but rather in the hormones that adult homosexuals had been exposed to while still in their mothers' wombs. This research continues on an ever grander scale, involving many millions of dollars, prestigious institutions, top-ranked journals in numerous specialties, and much more.

It all started humbly enough, with guinea pigs. In 1959, a scientific paper was published out of the University of Kansas titled "Organizing Action of Prenatally Administered Testosterone Propionate on the Tissues Mediating Mating Behavior in the Female Guinea Pig."[2] The research team exposed female guinea pig fetuses to so much testosterone that they were born with male-typical genitalia. Once these animals matured, they were tested for their response to further administration of androgens and estrogens. The team claimed that the results showed that prenatal hormone exposure has "an organizing or differentiating action on the neural tissues mediating mating behavior," while exposure to the same chemicals later in life "activates" the kind of mating behavior that was "organized" into the brain prenatally. This was the first formulation of what would become known as the organization/activation hypothesis.

The Ironies of (Dr.) Money

Here the story takes a sharp turn into terrain that is anything but humble, where we meet another supremely confident man of medicine, in this case not a medical doctor but a psychologist by the name of John Money. Raised in New Zealand, trained at Harvard, Dr. Money was adept at building the grandest of theories from the most meager data. He was respected and despised in equal measure, though never by the same person. As he commanded considerable persuasive powers, after polarizing the field in which he was working, his position would almost always carry the day. Until it all came crashing down.

Today, Money is mostly remembered as the creator and chief proselytizer of a protocol of intersex health care that dominated the field from the 1960s to the 1990s before falling into disgrace. ("Intersex" is a general term used for a variety of conditions in which a person is born with a reproductive or sexual anatomy that doesn't seem to fit the typical definitions of female or male.) Beyond that, Money is known as the man who led the fight for the right of transexuals (the word *transgender* had not yet been invented) to obtain hormone therapy and surgery in the United States. Surprisingly, his position as the progenitor of the contemporary theory of how the human brain is sexed is largely forgotten.

This is one of the many ironies of John Money. In *clinical practice,* the premise of the approach to intersex health care that Money tirelessly championed was his claim that what he called "psychosexual differentiation" ("gender identity" in today's terminology) is a social phenomenon instilled during the earliest years of life by child rearing and environment. Yet his *research* launched the school of thought that asserts the opposite: that when it comes to the source of gender identity, prenatal hormones—not child rearing and environment—trump all.

Money got his PhD from Harvard and went immediately to Johns Hopkins University, where he became part of a small group of clinicians with a specialty practice in what are now called intersex conditions. Since visual examination of such children at birth may not yield an immediate designation of "male" or "female," individual intersex children may be raised in very different gender regimens. One particular disorder can result in a child who appears female at birth and is thus raised as a girl until facial hair and a lowered voice arrive with puberty. At that point further investigation reveals the presence of undescended testicles and male-type chromosomes, and the teenager often switches from living as female to male.

The process of the differentiation of fetal genitalia into male or female type is considered well understood, and is regulated by fetal exposure to androgens and estrogens in the womb. Thus, intersex disorders are hormonal.

In his 1952 dissertation, Money examined the relation of intersex patients' gender identity (or sense of themselves as being male or female) to their physiology, and found nothing in their bodies that consistently correlated with their gender identity: not the visual appearance of their genitals, not the presence of ovaries or testicles, not male- or female-type chromosomes. The only variable that reliably predicted whether the intersex patient *felt* male or female was whether the child had been reared as a boy or a girl.[3] Eventually Money reasoned that gender identity is like one's first language: it is not set before birth but soon after, and once the deed is done it cannot be undone.

Money's conclusion had immediate implications for intersex care at Johns Hopkins and eventually around the nation. The profound anguish he witnessed among his intersex patients and their families convinced him that it was impossible to live happily as neither male nor female in the American culture of the time. Since his research showed that gender identity came not from the body but from rearing, Money reasoned that the best course of action was to surgically alter the patient's genitalia so as to appear as typically male or female as possible, and then raise the child as whichever sex the surgeon's knife had created. Since he believed that gender identity was indelibly imprinted at a very young age, the earlier the surgery and gender-specific child rearing could begin, the better the chances of a successful outcome (in this case, a successful outcome was a life in which the intersex condition was not a source of constant anguish). Practically, this resulted in most intersex children being raised as girls, since both doctors and parents found it inconceivable that a person could live happily as a man without a penis that could become erect and penetrate a vagina, and surgeons were far more adept at constructing something like a vagina than a penis.

Money was a quintessential medical crusader, and once convinced of this course of action, crusading he went, writing books and journal articles, traveling, cajoling, delivering lectures, and giving interviews, reshaping the medical standards of intersex care as he went.

Not surprisingly, Money's confidence in his own prescriptions was matched by the ferocity of the criticisms he received. To begin with, the surgeries were exceedingly painful, required long recoveries, and often resulted in loss of sensation and sexual function, as well as complications that could cause lifelong difficulties that required subsequent surgeries.

His parenting protocol came under even harsher attack from critics who pointed out that parents who followed his advice reinforced the most stereotypical gender norms. This was necessarily so, since the goal of the whole endeavor was to raise a child whose sense of self matched the prevailing expectations of who girls and boys were supposed to be. The closer the fit, the more successful the outcome. But this was all happening in the 1960s and 1970s, a time of unprecedented upheaval in precisely those gender norms. Men with long hair! Women in pants! Women's Liberation! Gay liberation! Women with careers! To his critics, Money's intersex protocol was a sexual counterrevolution dressed up with a phony air of medical authority. But here again we run into another of the deep ironies of Dr. Money: his "promise that biology was not destiny, and that females were socialized to be 'women,'" as *Time* magazine paraphrased him in 1973, resonated with the feminists of the day, who argued that women could do anything men could do and that the limited career options for women at the time were simply the result of men setting the rules. Money's research seemed to give Simone de Beauvoir's iconic feminist declaration that "one is not born, but rather becomes, a woman" the status of scientifically proven fact, but his clinical practice ran counter to everything feminists were trying to accomplish.[4]

Dr. Money's Flagship Case

Money had one case in particular that he referred to again and again in books, journal articles, lectures, and interviews, as proof that when it comes to gender, rearing trumps all.[5] He identified the patient as "John/Joan," a child whose penis had been severed in a botched circumcision. Under Money's guidance, surgery to remove the testicles was performed and the child was raised as a girl. Money reported that "Joan's" sense of herself as female was complete, and that she "preferred dresses to pants, enjoyed wearing her hair ribbons, bracelets, and frilly blouses, and loved being her Daddy's little sweetheart."[6]

One of Money's fiercest critics was a medical researcher named Milton Diamond, who had worked in the University of Kansas lab that had published the original findings on the mating behavior of female guinea pigs exposed prenatally to testosterone.[7] His subsequent animal research reaffirmed his conclusion that prenatal hormone exposure, not social experience, determined much about human gender behavior. Years later Diamond tracked down "John/Joan's" former psychiatrist. Together, the two men published an article in 1997 revealing that the patient, whose real name was David Reimer, had threatened suicide at age thirteen unless his parents would permit him to live as a boy, despite being unaware of his medical past.[8] His parents then revealed to him the story of the loss of his penis, and David immediately began living as a male. The journal article was followed by a BBC documentary, a *Rolling Stone* article, a seemingly endless series of academic books and articles, and in 2001 a book of David's life story told in the first person but written by John Colapinto, the journalist who covered the story for *Rolling Stone*.[9] Titled *As Nature Made Him: The Story of a Boy Who Was Raised as a Girl*, the book depicted Money as a terrifying medical monster and quickly became a best seller. The following year David's twin brother committed suicide. Two years later, David committed suicide as well.

Few medical careers have gone down in flames as spectacularly as that of John Money. During the height of the media hoopla concerning the Reimer case, virtually no one came to his defense. But once the smoke had cleared, it became apparent that nothing about intersex care had been resolved. Money and others favoring his approach could point to cases that seemingly succeeded just as dramatically as Reimer's had failed. What accounted for the different outcomes? The comparatively late age of Reimer's circumcision and change from boy to girl? Or did his parents balk at enforcing crucial gender norms during his upbringing? Depending on whose version of the story you listen to, the tragedy of David Reimer is either a tale of a brilliant doctor brought down by his rivals on the basis of one failed case, a tale of an arrogant megalomaniac who wrecked the lives of his suffering patients, or a tale of a terribly unfortunate young person whose penis was severed at a very early age and who was then used as a medical football by ambitious men on all sides until finally driven to suicide.

Money and Sex Reassignment Surgery

Before his fall from grace, Money's other major undertaking at Johns Hopkins was his Gender Identity Clinic, which opened in 1966. Sex reassignment surgeries for transexuals were unavailable in the United States at the time, and nearly unavailable anywhere else. Surgeries had been available through Hirschfeld's Institute for Sexual Science in Germany until the Nazis came to power, sacked the institute, and sent Hirschfeld into exile. Christine Jorgensen—a US Army soldier turned "blonde bombshell"—had become a national and international celebrity after convincing surgeons in Denmark to operate on her, but the Danes made clear that Jorgensen's case was not the beginning of a more general availability of such procedures in that country.[10]

The first sex reassignment surgery in the United States was performed on a patient known to the world by the pseudonym Agnes. Agnes appeared typically male at birth and went through childhood as a boy, but Agnes's body began to noticeably feminize during her teenage years, and at seventeen the youth switched to living as a girl. She had, in the words of her doctors, "large well-developed breasts" and male-type chromosomes and gonads. Doctors determined that the estrogen that was feminizing her body was being produced in atypically large quantities by her testicles, a condition they called Testicular Feminization Syndrome. In 1959 a team of surgeons removed the male genitalia and surgically constructed a vagina.

Soon after, David Lee Cameron had sex reassignment surgery at the Buffalo General Hospital. But Cameron turned around and filed a $5 million lawsuit (equivalent to $35 million in 2015) against his doctors and the hospital for performing the operation. Cameron claimed the doctors had made him into "a freak and nonentity, without sex or sexual reproduction organs" and had led him to believe he "would be cured of his previous psychological problems," a cure Cameron did not experience.[11] The suit was settled out of court for an undisclosed amount.

The Cameron lawsuit effectively ended sex reassignment surgery in the United States. Those who had read the extensive press coverage of Jorgensen and wanted such surgery for themselves had nowhere to turn. Many wrote to Jorgensen, who referred them to Harry Benjamin, who could offer them little more than a sympathetic letter in reply.

John Money set out to change that. In doing so, he worked closely with Benjamin and Reed Erickson. Born Rita Alma Erickson in El Paso in 1917, Erickson was the multimillionaire heir of a lead-smelting operation. Options were apparently available to someone of Erickson's means that were not widely available to others, and in the early 1960s Erickson obtained a hysterectomy in New York, a double mastectomy at Johns Hopkins, and a passport identifying him as Reed Erickson. He then founded the Erickson Educational Foundation, through which he channeled $50,000 to Benjamin and an even larger chunk of money to Money, which Money used to open the Gender Identity Clinic at Johns Hopkins in 1966. Monthly meetings of EEF grant recipients were held in Harry Benjamin's office, with Erickson, Benjamin, and Money in attendance.

Like the Johns Hopkins intersex care program, the Gender Identity Clinic was the work of Money, who "argued, cajoled, and arm-twisted reluctant colleagues into translating the expertise they had acquired treating intersexual people into treating transexuals."[12] The clinic performed ten surgeries in its first six months, and received major press coverage. *Time, Newsweek,* and many major dailies carried sensational accounts. Baltimore's Catholic Church even made a statement announcing that the Church had no objection.

In the wake of the Jorgensen sex-change sensation, heated debates similar to those at Johns Hopkins erupted at other major public health centers. When Money convinced Johns Hopkins to jump first and take the media glare, others quickly followed. Soon surgeries were being offered at Northwestern, then Stanford, then the University of Washington in Seattle, then others. By the end of the 1970s more than a thousand sex reassignment surgeries had been performed by doctors at universities across the country.[13]

All these programs were quickly overwhelmed with requests for far more surgeries than they could accommodate, and no method for deciding who among the applicants would be accepted. Psychiatrists at each institution were scathing in their criticisms of any surgeries at all, arguing that those requesting the surgeries were self-hating homosexuals who needed counseling more than surgery. Many surgeons voiced the same objection. Paul McHugh, the psychiatrist who led the charge against Money at Johns Hopkins, remembered, "The surgeons were saying to me, 'Imagine what it's like to get up in the morning and come in and hack away at perfectly normal organs because you psychiatrists don't know what to do with these people.'"[14]

For most types of surgery, priority is given to patients with the most dire diagnosis. If there is a line for a cancer surgery, the patient with the most advanced cancer goes first. But even those doctors supporting sex reassignment surgeries were having a hard time articulating diagnostic criteria. Whose case of Gender Identity Disorder was the most dire?

Doctors are sworn to, above all else, "do no harm." What was the pathology for which they were being asked to remove healthy organs? Wouldn't they get sued for that? Or banned from practicing surgery altogether? Was it even legal?

There ensued an encore performance of Magnus Hirschfeld's endless attempts to develop a nosology of gender pathology. Fifty years before, Hirschfeld had finally settled on four types of "sexual intermediaries": hermaphrodites, androgynes, transvestites, and homosexuals. Now Money and his colleagues set about distinguishing "genuine transexuals" from "pseudo transexuals" and so on. Failing to establish a stable diagnostic framework, Benjamin suggested that the diagnosis required for the surgery could be the request for the surgery itself, arguing that anyone who was sick enough to ask for such painful, ferocious surgery was sick enough to receive it.[15] Not surprisingly, this proposal convinced no one.

Much of the debate boiled down to whether the requests for surgery resulted from a psychiatric or a hormonal disorder. Those on both sides of the debate clung fervently to their position despite there being no evidence for either. The empty-handed search for the alleged hormonal imbalance that resulted in requests for sex reassignment surgery on the one hand was matched on the other by psychiatrists' inability to explain how life experiences might lead to such a request, and psychiatrists' failure to produce a single patient who was "cured" of a desire for surgery through psychiatric means. As the historian Joanne Meyerowitz has noted, it was this debate that catapulted the concept of *gender* onto center stage:

> The concept of gender was widely adopted, in part perhaps because it did not preclude opposing visions of etiology. The gender identity might result from hormones or genes or brain structure, from imprinting or conditioning or other forms of social learning, or from the psychodynamic processes of identification during mother-infant interaction. Participants on all sides of the debate could use the language of gender without undermining their favored position. Gender, then came to dominate the scientific approach to transexuality, but it did not resolve the debates about the causes.[16]

Robert Stoller, Harold Garfinkel, and Agnes

For seven years, the hormonal-disorder advocates had one star exhibit in their corner: Agnes, the nation's first recipient of sex reassignment surgery. Since her condition was so unusual—male chromosomes, fully developed male genitalia, and female breasts—she had been the subject of exhaustive medical testing prior to approval for surgery, including an abdominal laparotomy (exploratory surgery), bilateral testicular biopsies, x-ray examinations of the chest and skull, a buccal smear, a urethral smear, a skin biopsy, and an extraordinary array of laboratory tests on her blood and urine.[17] She was extensively interviewed at UCLA by Dr. Robert Stoller, a psychiatrist, and Harold Garfinkel, a sociologist. Agnes never wavered from her insistence that humans do *not* exist on a spectrum of gender, that all humans are male or female, with no in between, and she was the latter. She flatly rejected any suggestion that she was homosexual or transexual, and refused to even meet such patients.

Stoller was to UCLA what Money was to Johns Hopkins: a psychiatrist working in an endocrinology unit with intersex patients, and a firm believer that those requesting sex reassignment surgery suffered from a hormonal imbalance.[18] For Stoller, Agnes was his smoking gun, a patient with an obvious biological force impelling her from male to female. That source had a diagnosis: Testicular Feminization Syndrome, or "a diffuse lesion of the testis [that is] the source of the feminizing effect."[19] Shortly after the testes were removed, doctors diagnosed Agnes with menopause, which confirmed their diagnosis that the testes had indeed been the source of the feminizing estrogens. The testes were sent to experts in other medical centers, who confirmed them as capable of producing Testicular Feminization Syndrome.[20]

For his part, Garfinkel was busy formulating his theory of "ethnomethodology," which he hoped would secure him a position in the pantheon of American sociologists as the peer of his Harvard professor, Talcott Parsons. Ethnomethodology is "the study of the everyday methods that people use for the production of social order."[21] With the arrival of a patient who would willingly sit for hours at a time over a period of months reciting the hypervigilant "everyday methods" she had employed over many years to fully comply with every conceivable female gender norm, as well as the terrible anxiety she experienced when her rigid enactment of femaleness failed to convince others, Garfinkel had hit pay dirt.[22]

In her encounter with UCLA, Agnes thus landed in not one but two independent fields of scholarship in which hers was the holy grail of case studies. What the John/Joan case became for intersex care, the Agnes case became to both ethnomethodology and the newly emerging field of transexual care. Importantly for the doctors trying to push a radical new kind of surgery through notoriously cautious medical institutions, Agnes was a perfect patient. Garfinkel's published description of her provides a clear picture of what doctors and scholars of the late 1950s expected from a patient who qualified for sex reassignment surgery:

> She was tall, slim, with a very female shape. Her measurements were 38-25-38. She had long, fine dark-blonde hair, a young face with pretty features, a peaches-and-cream complexion, no facial hair, subtly plucked eyebrows, and no makeup except for lipstick. At the time of her first appearance she was dressed in a tight sweater which marked off her thin shoulders, ample breasts, and narrow waist. . . . There was nothing garish or exhibitionistic in her attire, nor was there any hint of poor taste or that she was ill at ease in her clothing, as is seen so frequently in transvestites and in women with disturbances in sexual identification. Her voice, pitched at an alto level, was soft, and her delivery had the occasional lisp similar to that affected by feminine appearing male ho-

mosexuals. Her manner was appropriately feminine with a slight awkwardness that is typical of middle adolescence.[23]

Both doctors published extensively on the case. Stoller published in the *Journal of Clinical Endocrinology and Metabolism,* and presented the case at the 1963 International Psychoanalytic Congress in Stockholm.[24] Garfinkel devoted an extensive chapter to Agnes in his 1967 book, *Studies in Ethnomethodology.*

But in 1966, the very year Money opened the Gender Identity Clinic at Johns Hopkins, Agnes confessed that she had actually been a hormonally typical boy who from age twelve had taken estrogen pills pilfered from his mother's post-hysterectomy estrogen prescription.

So much for the smoking gun.

The revelation was a major embarrassment not only to Stoller and Garfinkel but to UCLA. Stoller was compelled to retract his findings and publish a *mea culpa.* Garfinkel learned of these developments while his book was in press, and had to rush a hastily written and highly embarrassing insert into his chapter on Agnes.

Nevertheless the hormones-determine-gender camp held steady to their course. Richard Green, the founding editor of the *Archives of Sexual Behavior,* coeditor with John Money of *Transsexualism and Sex Reassignment* (published by Johns Hopkins University Press in 1969), and later founder and president of the Harry Benjamin International Gender Dysphoria Association, advised his colleagues, "Do not despair about the biological force behind gender identity. I am sure there is one somewhere."[25]

"Problems That Don't Go Away"

As the 1960s turned to the 1970s, clinics offering sex reassignment surgery and hormone therapy for transexuals appeared increasingly out of step with the times. In 1969, New York City police raided a gay bar called the Stonewall Inn, setting off extended rioting in the West Village. The Gay Liberation Front formed soon after. The tenor of the sexual subculture leaned more toward marching in the street and fighting cops than checking into the hospital for hormones and surgery. That same year Barbara Seaman's *The Doctors' Case against the Pill* became a bestseller. The following year members of D.C. Women's Liberation created a media sensation by disrupting the Senate hearings on the Pill. Second-wave feminism was finding its voice in the strident rejection of the marketing campaigns mounted by giant pharmaceutical corporations selling the idea that femininity equaled estrogen, and that estrogen was safe. Sylvester rocketed out of San Francisco's gay underground to become an international disco icon, appearing at times as male, at other times female, but most times a flamboyant mix of both. When asked what gay liberation meant to him, Sylvester replied that it meant that "I could be the queen that I really was without having a sex change or being on hormones."[26]

In 1974 the controversy over Money's Gender Identity Clinic that had long simmered behind closed doors at Johns Hopkins erupted into public. A Johns Hopkins psychoanalyst, Jon K. Meyer, coauthored a paper attacking Money's clinic, charging that the care the clinic offered merely "seems to temporarily palliate an unfortunate emotional state, rather than really cure the problem."[27] The following year Stoller, still smarting from the Agnes affair, told a symposium at the American Medical Association, "The level of discourse on transsexualism stinks."[28]

Since no one agreed on what "the problem" was, there was no agreement on how to define a "cure." Surgeons typically measure a surgery's success or failure by *outcome*. In many kinds of surgery, measuring outcome means determining whether those who received surgery outlive those who did not. How might one measure the outcome, in this sense of the word, for sex reassignment surgery? By how well the patient conformed to the social expectations of the new gender? Critics charged that this measure only reinforced gender stereotypes. By the number of patients who discontinued psychiatric treatment? Wouldn't that discourage people who needed treatment from seeking it? By how many patients got jobs and stayed out of jail? But wouldn't that impose a class bias in favor of well-to-do patients? By whether the patients themselves said they were happier? But this was surgery, not psychiatry. Surgeries that are are not intended to cure a disease and are undertaken solely for the happiness of the patient are deemed cosmetic, and are not covered by health insurance.

In 1977, Meyer coauthored a study of sex reassignment surgery outcomes that answered none of these questions to anyone's satisfaction. In 1979 he called a press conference to publicize his study, telling the *New*

York Times, "Surgery is not a proper treatment for a psychiatric disorder, and it's clear to me that these patients have severe psychological problems that don't go away after surgery."[29] He referred to one particular case in which a post-op female-to-male required hospitalization for drug dependency and suicidal intention. That person was likely Reed Erickson, the heir to the lead-smelting fortune who had funded the Johns Hopkins Gender Identity Clinic, and who had checked into the Johns Hopkins psychiatric clinic for "psychosis with drug intoxication," the start of an extended decline through drug addiction, paranoia, and delusion that lasted until his death in 1992.

The Gender Identity Clinic at Johns Hopkins was closed in 1979. Similar clinics at other universities followed suit. Some imploded as a result of similar controversies. Others, like the clinic at Stanford, did not actually close but simply moved off the campus and went private.[30] Surgeons at private clinics did not have to justify their practice to university boards. And they could make a lot of money performing surgeries that university hospitals denied.

7

Brain Organization Theory

Though both his intersex and transexual clinical practices crumbled around him, the ideas on which John Money based those practices have had far more staying power. Indeed, they have come to dominate thinking about hormones and gender, despite having no more evidence supporting them now they had in 1960.

One of the very first problems Money's ideas encountered was the 1959 guinea pig research from Kansas, which stimulated a wave of follow-up studies that seemed to support the original study's conclusion that prenatal hormone exposure "organized" mammal brains into male and female types, which were "activated" later by postnatal hormone exposure (typically puberty). As this research accumulated, it posed an increasingly pointed challenge to Money's assertion that gendered behavior in humans was determined socially soon after birth.

In 1965 Money published a review of thirty-six recent animal studies and tried to reconcile them with his own research. Reviewing his own data, Money now claimed to have indeed found certain "masculinized" behaviors among women with congenital adrenal hyperplasia, a particular intersex disorder known to involve atypically heavy prenatal exposure to androgens. The difference, Money explained, could be measured in how these women experienced sexual "arousal." Some women with atypically high prenatal androgen exposure, he reported, were more aroused by "visual and narrative perceptual material" than other women. What was more, their sexual arousal was more intense, "more than the ordinary woman's arousal of romantic feeling and desire to be with her husband or boy friend."[1]

Two years later Money published again, this time with Anke Ehrhardt, a PhD student working under him at Johns Hopkins. Their study involved observation of the behavior of ten girls with intersexual disorders involving prenatal exposure to progestin. It was the first study to examine human behavior in light of the new ideas emerging from animal research about the "organizing" effect of prenatal hormone exposure on the brain. Here again, Money reported that these girls had been prenatally masculinized as measured by their IQs, which were higher than expected for girls. The belief that women score lower than men on IQ tests has since been refuted, but research based on that assumption continues even today to be cited as evidence of how prenatal hormones sex the brain. This is an early example of a core problem that continues to plague such brain organization research down to the present day: evidence of the sexual differentiation of brains is measured according to the prevailing gender norms of the day, which then go out of date, yet the research continues to be cited as valid.[2]

Over the next six years, Ehrhardt and Money were a whirlwind of publishing, producing more than two new research reports every year, as well as a book, *Man and Woman, Boy and Girl,* published in 1972, that put them in the public eye.[3] Each report found that high levels of prenatal androgen exposure had "masculinized" one aspect or another of female behavior, while low levels of prenatal androgen exposure had "feminized" one aspect or another of male behavior. Variables they measured included verbal and math ability, the kinds of careers their subjects were interested in, and "marriage and motherhood" (lower than "expected" interest in marriage indicated a "masculinized" woman).

Intersex conditions are relatively rare, so Ehrhardt and Money had only a few subjects whose behavior they could observe. In fact, the subjects in many of these studies were the very same individuals who had been the subjects of Money's earlier work. In other words, he studied the same group of people at two different times, concluding the first time that their behavior demonstrated that gender and sexuality were entirely determined by socialization, and the second time that their behavior indicated aspects of gender and sexuality were determined by prenatal hormone exposure. What changed between the first study and the second was the researchers' expectations, which had been reshaped by the appearance of a theory of how prenatal hormones "organize" the brain.[4]

No one else was doing brain organization research in humans during these years, so by the time others arrived in the field they found it already populated by more than a dozen papers and a book, all by Money and his junior colleagues. And his papers continued to pile up for decades hence. But by the 1970s, Money had company in the field. A lot of company.

Brain Organization Theory and LGBT Politics

Today the hunt for the source of homosexuality, gender identity, and indeed all "masculinity" and "femininity" in the brain has become a truly colossal enterprise, on a far grander scale than ever attained by the search for the source of the same phenomena in the gonads. Steinach and Hirschfeld would be stunned. Many millions of dollars have been spent. Strange behaviors and deformities have been produced in laboratory animals of all sorts. Children have been observed, brains dissected, electronic sensors attached to penises, databases constructed, numbers crunched, conferences attended, careers advanced, and honors bestowed. An enormous body of research has accumulated, which sprawls across many sciences, specialties, journals, and institutions.

By the time Rebecca M. Jordan-Young set out to do the first and only systematic review of the literature, which she published in 2011, there were over three hundred published, peer-reviewed research papers, each citing others which cited others. And they continue to accumulate at an accelerating rate: since the first paper in the 1950s, each successive decade has seen more papers published than the preceding one.[5] The influence of this research on contemporary culture is profound. Research results are rushed from the pages of scientific journals to the front pages of the *New York Times* and *Time,* public radio, network television, and best-selling books. Often, the tentative research findings of the scientific journals arrive in the public square dressed up as fact. As Jordan-Young notes:

> The notion that there are male brains and female brains has continued to crop up in controversies over women in math and science, but it has also recently shown up in discussions of single-sex education, sex disparities in wages, "abstinence-only" sexuality education curricula,

the protocol for medical treatment of children born with ambiguous genitalia, and yes, even the out-of-control, risky trading that recently brought the economy to its knees [in 2008]. . . . In an era where diversity is celebrated, the idea of "sex in the brain" no longer equals an endorsement of male superiority, and critics of the idea are increasingly cast as not only antiscience, but antidiversity.[6]

While the notion of innately different preferences in men and women was once politically suspect, it is now often suggested that accepting these innate differences will encourage a more rational approach to equality. Should boys and girls be taught differently, because the sexes have innately different patterns of learning? Perhaps we should stop striving for parity in the professions, for example, or for an equal division of parenting labor, because women and men want different things out of life and are temperamentally suited both for different work and for a different balance between career and family.[7]

One reason the theory has captured the popular imagination so effectively is the enthusiastic embrace it has received in the LGBT community. The theory asserts that the same process that differentiates male brains from female brains also differentiates homosexual brains from heterosexual brains. The stubborn feeling of being of a "female soul in a male body" and vice versa has been voiced for at least 150 years. When the phrase first appeared in print in 1865, the term *homosexual* had not even been coined.[8] The feeling has persisted down through the decades despite a complete lack of physical evidence as to why this should be so, and in the face of a terrifying assortment of punishments intended to eradicate it. Now, in the twenty-first century, at long last science seemed to vindicate what so many had seemingly known from personal experience. Of course, few people talk of the "soul" these days. Today it is not a female soul that has mistakenly taken up residence in a male body but a female brain.

The LGBT community has political reasons for embracing brain organization theory as well, since the theory removes the source of sexual nonconformity from the realms of moral failing or willpower and moves it squarely into the realm of biology. Here the modern LGBT community has followed the same path trod by Magnus Hirschfeld, who championed Steinach's discovery of "F-cells" in homosexual testicles as indisputably settled science for the exact same reason.

Tragically, the belief that sexual deviance is biological did not confer on sexual minorities in Hitler's Germany the protections Hirschfeld anticipated. When the Nazis came to power, the idea that sexual minorities were "born that way" and could not be changed became the rationale for rounding them up and putting them in concentration camps.

Brain organization theory has an additional, very particular importance for the transgender wing of the LGBT community. Winning access to surgery and hormone therapy—which are both expensive and only legally available with a doctor's approval—has been a central concern of transgender activism. In the United States, perhaps no issue has been of greater priority to activists. Their case is helped enormously by the assertion that there really is such a thing as a male brain in a female body and vice versa, and that this is determined by prenatal hormone exposure. Activists can point out that other maladies resulting from prenatal hormone pathologies are covered by insurance—so why should this particular one be denied?

The high political stakes attached to brain organization theory were what motivated Rebecca Jordan-Young to spend years doing the first and only systematic analysis of the more than three hundred studies "on the ostensible prenatal hormone-sexuality connection published from 1967, when the theory was first applied to humans, up to the year 2000, when the increased flow of research in this area made it no longer possible to examine every published study in depth."[9] That no one had ever done such a thing should raise some basic questions about how scientific research is done in an era when far more studies are published each year than ever before. Here was a huge mass of interconnected research done over several decades; each study cited many others whose results bolstered its findings, and the cited studies cited still others, which often created a chain that would loop back around to the first study.

But this is how scientific research is supposed to work, isn't it? A critical mass of scientists prioritize the same research, research funds appear as a result, the heads of various labs propose their own unique approach to the problem, the money is distributed, and everyone gets to work. Researchers then submit their results to their scientific peers, who verify that the results have been obtained using correct scientific method, and the results are then published and compared to the published, peer-reviewed results of other labs. At the end of the day, if everybody is citing lots of other studies that corroborate their results, then scientific knowledge is being produced, right?

Brain Organization Theory Basics

The hypothesis at the center of all this activity is fairly simple: the same mechanisms that cause fetal genitalia to differentiate into male and female also cause fetal brains to differentiate into male and female. In both cases, the determining factors are the estrogens and androgens the fetus is exposed to in utero. In the words of the initial paper's authors, "the rules of hormonal action are identical" whether the object of differential development is the brain or the genitals.[10]

"Sex hormones" still determine who becomes homosexual or transgender, but the decisive hormones are not in the blood of the individual but the womb of the individual's mother. Hormone exposure later in life—either endogenously from the body's own glands or exogenously from the world outside—can only "activate" behavioral predispositions that were "organized" into the fetal brain while in the womb. Thus the term "organization-activation hypothesis."

That's the theory. Pretty straightforward when it comes down to it.

The theory has the advantage of neatly explaining away decades of research showing that postnatal hormone exposures produce erratic, unpredictable results that cannot be reconciled with the anticipated results of something named a "sex hormone," no matter how diligently researchers futz with the numbers. The argument is that the reason exposing humans and animals to estrogen and testosterone produces such unpredictable results is that their brains were "organized" differently before they were born.

How would one go about proving or disproving this theory? If the research is to be judged by the same standards as, say, the research pharmaceutical companies are required to complete before marketing prescription drugs, a huge group of women would have to be recruited. These women would all be impregnated and then randomly assigned to receive one of many specific hormone exposures or placebos. There would have to be all kinds of different doses, administered at different times during pregnancy. Then the offsprings' behavior would have to be monitored for many years while keeping their experiences of the world identical and environments constant. Each one of these steps is either impossible or unethical. But this is what we ask of drug companies before we believe their claims about what chemicals do in the body.

Let's not forget that prescription drugs are often discovered to be inefficacious or harmful only *after* they are approved for public use. In other words, chemists often come up with theories that pass the kinds of rigorous tests brain organization theory cannot be subjected to, and they *still* turn out to be fallacious. But the fallacies cannot be uncovered by the procedures used to approve prescription drugs. The only way scientists have been able to identify these fallacies is to put the drugs on the market on a large scale and see what problems arise.

Since they are unable to subject their hypothesis to human experiment, brain organization theory researchers have pursued three alternatives. One is to find human babies known to have been exposed to atypically high or low prenatal androgen or estrogen levels and measure the masculinity or femininity of their behavior as they age. The second alternative is to begin with a group of adults who exhibit atypical gender behavior and work backward, trying to reconstruct what their prenatal hormonal milieus might have been. The third option is to experiment with animals, because they can be submitted to nightmarish procedures ruled unethical when performed on humans, often gestate and mature much faster than humans, and can be confined to (sort of) identical lab environments.

That's it for options, and each of those three-hundred-plus studies Jordan-Young reviewed used one or another of them. In practice, researchers pursuing the first alternative (starting with atypical fetal hormone levels and working forward) have studied either people known to have been prenatally exposed to some exogenous hormone (a hormone that entered the womb from outside the mother's body) or infants diagnosed with hormonal disorders known to result from fetal exposure to atypical amounts of endogenous hormones. Researchers pursing the second alternative (beginning with atypical gender behavior and working backward) have studied gays, lesbians, and the transgendered.

The hormonal disorders that have attracted the most research are congenital adrenal hyperplasia (CAH) and 5-alpha reductase deficiency (5-ARD). CAH is a genetic disorder that affects the adrenal glands, causing them to secrete androgens in larger quantities than is typical.

Infants born with this disorder require lifelong medication and suffer a range of effects that in extreme cases are fatal. Female infants with CAH may have genitalia closer in appearance to what is typically male than female. This form of CAH is thus considered an "intersex disorder," and it is the most common cause of genital ambiguity. Brain organization theory predicts that the high prenatal androgen exposure experienced by genetic females with CAH will result in women who are more likely to be homosexual, transgender, or transexual, and more masculine in behavior, than other women. Thus, the behavior of women with this disorder was the subject of John Money's first published papers, and of many others since.

In the case of 5-ARD, androgens are present in typical amounts during fetal development but an enzyme necessary for male genital development is absent, so genetic males with 5-ARD may be born with genitals that appear more female than male, and thus assumed to be baby girls until adolescence, when the testosterone their body produces causes their voices to lower, muscle mass to increase, and facial hair to appear. Since the prenatal hormone exposure of genetic males with 5-ARD is male-typical, brain organization theory predicts that these individuals will have "masculinized" brains in spite of being raised as girls. Children with 5-ARD make even more promising research subjects than children with classic CAH, because parents of girls with CAH are aware of their child's diagnosis, while parents of genetic males with 5-ARD are often completely unaware they are not raising a "real girl" until adolescence, and their parenting is thus assumed not to differ from the parenting of other girls.

Research on people known to have been prenatally exposed to exogenous hormones has focused on children of mothers given DES during pregnancy. DES, you may recall, was the first mass-marketed synthetic estrogen, and was given to up to 2 million pregnant women in the mistaken belief that it would reduce the risk of miscarriage. Instead, it was linked to rare cancers and other disorders. DES sales collapsed under a deluge of lawsuits, and registries of DES children were established to track the health of those affected. Here was something close to a ready-made brain-organization experiment: a very large group of pregnant women who had been deliberately administered synthetic "sex hormones," and large numbers of their offspring who were already being tracked by medical researchers.

Those pursuing the third research option, experimenting with animals, have used a variety of subjects. All together, rats, guinea pigs, sheep, vervet monkeys, genetic females with classic CAH, genetic males with 5-ARD, and DES daughters and sons have provided the raw material for scientists studying brain organization theory.

There are major problems, however, with each approach. Let's begin with animal studies. Genital differentiation in mammals is considered to be well understood, and the process is very similar across species, so making inferences about genital differentiation in humans from the results of studies of genital differentiation in rats is considered a safe bet. Brains are another matter entirely. The brains of guinea pigs, rats, and humans are not nearly as similar as their penises and vaginas. Humans are unique in how early in development babies are born compared to how long their brains continue to develop. Thus, at a comparable stage of brain development, a guinea pig would be isolated in the womb while a human would be in intense social interaction with other humans. If, that is, guinea pig and human brains develop in stages that are comparable. Would research that demonstrated how prenatal hormone exposure differentiates a "masculine" rat brain from a "female" rat brain tell us much that would be relevant to humans? And what would constitute masculine, feminine, homosexual, or transgender behavior in a guinea pig or, say, a vervet monkey?

For that matter, what constitutes masculine, feminine, homosexual, or transgender behavior in a *human*? Recall the account at the outset of this book of how vitriolic the debate about who is and is not transgender has become within the transgender community itself—a debate so intractable that the transgender historian Susan Stryker concluded that "there is no way of using the word [transgender] that doesn't offend some people by including them where they don't want to be included or excluding them from where they want to be included."[11] But the methodology of these studies requires that behaviors be precisely quantified. *How would you know who to count?*

Have the neuroendocrinologists discovered something Stryker missed? There are, after all, over three hundred peer-reviewed papers on the topic. Surely at least some of these scientists rigorously addressed these obstacles.

Jordan-Young's Symmetry Analysis

Technically speaking, Rebecca Jordan-Young did a *symmetry analysis* of more than three hundred studies. Symmetry analysis is what scientists do if they want to know whether different studies that address the same phenomenon yield results that are mutually supportive or mutually contradictory. A full discussion of the details of symmetry analysis would fill many pages, but the essential idea can be easily stated. For studies to be symmetrical, their *inputs* and *outputs* must be *consonant*. In the case of brain organization theory, the inputs are androgens and estrogens, and the outputs are masculine or feminine behavior. The definition of estrogens and androgens is pretty clear-cut, so most brain organization theory studies have symmetrical inputs. The outputs—masculine or feminine behavior—are another matter. Unless studies use the same definitions of masculine and feminine behavior, they are asymmetrical and their findings cannot be considered mutually supportive.

It is not enough that inputs and outputs are symmetrical; the *relationship* between inputs and outputs must also be consonant across studies. For example, two studies that use symmetrical inputs and outputs may show that variations in a given input produce variation in a given output, but if the *direction of change* in one study is opposite the direction of change in the other, the studies are contradictory. For example, two studies that examine the relationship between prenatal androgen exposure and masculine behavior in women might use the same definitions of prenatal androgen exposure and masculine behavior in women, and make the same claim that prenatal androgen exposure influences adult behavior. But if the results of one study show an increase in masculine behavior and the other a decrease, the studies not only fail to support each other but are actually contradictory.

By rigorously limiting her review to the symmetry of the research, Jordan-Young evaluated the science of brain organization theory on its own terms and at face value. In brief, the question that she asked was, "Are these studies even logical in their reasoning?"

What she found is a stunning indictment of an entire field of present-day scientific endeavor.

To begin with, the outputs are often asymmetrical to the point of absurdity. For example, many studies have searched for signs of "mas-

culinization" in the toy preferences of girls with CAH. A frequent criticism of this work is that it cannot discern whether these preferences are
acquired during childhood or inscribed on the brain before birth. In
response, one 2002 study looked at toy preferences in vervet monkeys,
reasoning that monkeys are not socialized to be "boys" and "girls." The
researchers thus measured the amount of time male and female monkeys spent playing with a cooking pot and a toy police car. But monkeys
don't watch their mothers cook or dream of the thrill of driving a car
with an emergency light and siren when they grow up.[12]

When examining women instead of monkeys, "masculinization" has
been measured by how often a woman initiates sex with her partner, how
much she enjoys "experimenting in sexual foreplay," her "variety of positions in sexual intercourse rather than just one or two," how much she
masturbates, and her interest in a career and life outside the home of a
nuclear family. I trust many female readers will be startled to learn just
how "masculinized" prenatal androgen exposure has made their brains.[13]

Beyond such absurdities, Jordan-Young found that when she put all
the studies together and compared inputs and outputs, the entire body
of research collapsed in an asymmetrical heap. In other words, even
if every measure of "masculinization" and "feminization" used in the
research is accepted as valid, the field is riddled with studies that cite
studies that cite more studies, all claiming their measurements match
when in fact they measure completely different things. In particular,
Jordan-Young discovered an across-the-board change in measurements
that occurred around 1980, when many behaviors previously coded as
feminine became gender-neutral. For example, having multiple sexual
partners and more varied and frequent sexual activities changed from
counting as prenatal masculinization to counting as typical female sexuality. At about the same time, the weight accorded to sexual orientation
increased substantially. In other words, far from tracking some deep
biological process, the field simply mirrored the changes in sexual behavior resulting from the social revolutions of the 1960s and 1970s, when
women's sexual lives were becoming more varied and gays and lesbians
more visible.

The consequences for the rigor of the research are catastrophic. When
Jordan-Young systematically worked through the implications of these
changes, item by item and study by study, she found that "studies showing a link between androgens and *masculinized* sexuality in the second

period are showing a link between androgens and *feminine* sexuality, according to the definitions used in the first period."[14] Yet studies from the later period continued to cite earlier studies as corroborating their findings.

Amazingly, after interviewing many of the top scientists in the field, Jordan-Young concluded that there was no deliberate fraud in all this: *no one noticed that what they were measuring had changed.*

The field is riddled with another problem with even more serious consequences. Enormous weight is given to sexual orientation in many studies, and it is worth taking the time to explain why. Remember that brain organization theory asserts that the same processes produce sexual differentiation in both the genitals and the brain. Imagine putting a bunch of humans in a big pile and then sorting them into male and female by looking at their genitals. The resulting piles would make a very accurate division. Yes, there would be some intersex people who would confound the process, but everyone would agree that the large majority of people had ended up in the right piles. Now put those same people back into a pile and divide them into male and female by asking them who graduated from college. We would not have one pile of men and one pile of women with a few confounding cases. We would have a big mess, because even if we had done this during the first two decades of brain organization research, when more males than females actually did graduate from college, the discrepancy was not so large that males and females could be reliably sorted based on college attendance. And if we had done the division today, when more women than men graduate from college (to such an extent that hand-wringing over how higher education might become more welcoming to males is a frequent topic of discussion in certain academic circles), we would have more women than men in the male pile.

Now imagine putting everyone back into a big pile and sorting again, putting those whose sexual partners were male in one pile and those whose sexual partners were female in the other. Our piles would be relatively well-sorted. Not nearly as well-sorted as when we sorted by genital appearance, because the number of people in the United States with same-sex attraction is by all counts much greater than the number with ambiguous genitalia. But the piles that resulted from sorting by sexual orientation would have more people in the right piles than any other behavioral measure that has been tested. In other words, if you are looking for a measure of human *behavior* that can reliably distinguish male from female, the sex of sexual partners is your best bet. Most women can be reliably predicted to have only male sexual partners, and most men can be reliably predicted to have only female sexual partners.

This is why brain organization researchers have an insatiable appetite for observing the most trivial details of the behavior of gays and lesbians.

But here we are right back at the *how would you know who to count?* problem. Can we accurately measure who is gay or lesbian any better than we can count who is transgender? For studies to be symmetrical, the measurement of homosexuality must be rigorously uniform across studies. So, precisely what behavior makes a person homosexual? Does just one sexual liaison with a male partner put a male research subject in the "feminized" pile? How about two? Three? How about one in college and nothing else since? When Jordan-Young asked the leading brain organization researchers these questions, she was repeatedly told that masculine and feminine sexuality are simply "commonsense" ideas. As one scientist said, "Most people . . . don't have any problem understanding that male sexuality is different from female sexuality. It's a no-brainer."[15]

John Money, the founding father of the field, explained that his answer to this problem rested on the difference between an "act" and a "status":

> The Skyscraper Test exemplifies the difference between act and status. One of the versions of this test applies to a person with a homosexual status who is atop the Empire State Building or other high building and is pushed to the edge of the parapet by a gun-toting, crazed sex terrorist with a heterosexual status. Suppose the homosexual is a man and the terrorist a woman who demands that he perform oral sex with her or go over the edge. To save his life, he might do it. If so, he would have performed a heterosexual act, but he would not have changed to have a heterosexual status.[16]

Good to have that cleared up.

Contradictory Frames of Sexual Orientation

Let's *pretend* for a moment that homosexuality has both a definition on which we can all agree and a measurement that can reliably indicate the quantity of its presence or absence. Now the methodological problems that pervade studies claiming to link prenatal hormones with homosexuality become even worse, because their inputs (prenatal hormone exposure) and outputs (homosexuality) would be consonant but the relationship between them would be contradictory. The reasoning here is something of a brain teaser, but it is worthwhile to work it through because the problem is endemic among brain organization studies.[17]

To illustrate, consider two studies, A and B. Both claim to have found a correlation between prenatal androgen exposure and homosexuality, and each research group cites the other's findings as corroborating. Study A found correlations between high androgen exposure and attraction to women, and low androgen exposure and attraction to men. Thus high androgen exposure correlated with lesbians and straight men, and low androgen exposure correlated with straight women and gay men. The study's authors report their conclusion that androgen exposure causes homosexuality.

But Study B correlated high androgen exposure with same-sex attraction, and low androgen exposure with opposite-sex attraction. Thus high androgen exposure correlated with homosexuality in both men and women, and low androgen exposure with heterosexuality in both men and women. The study's authors announce that their results confirm Study A's conclusion that androgen exposure causes homosexuality.

This is the trick that allows two studies to be presented as mutually supporting a connection between androgen exposure and homosexuality, even though one shows that male homosexuality *increases* with greater prenatal androgen exposure, and the other study shows that male homosexuality *decreases* with greater prenatal androgen exposure. The studies are thus contradictory. Even if both studies measure homosexuality precisely the same way, at least one of the studies *must* be wrong.

Animal studies make the whole mess even messier, as they often correlate hormone exposure not to desire for males or females, nor to desire for the same or opposite sex, but to desire to sexually penetrate or be penetrated. Whether the partner is male or female, or of the same or opposite sex as the subject, is not considered relevant. For example, many rat studies classify male rats who allow other males to mount them as "homosexual," but not the male rats doing the mounting. These studies echo the way human male homosexuality was socially understood in the United States before World War II, when the big taboo for men was allowing sexual penetration by another man, not sexually penetrating

another man. The act of being penetrated marked the loss of one's manhood. The manhood of the men doing the penetrating was considered
confirmed and even elevated by their prowess at sexually penetrating
both men and women. This understanding of homosexuality continues
to be the principle dividing line of acceptable and unacceptable male
sexual behavior in some parts of the world.[18] It has all but disappeared in
the United States today, except in studies of brain organization theory
that use lab animals.

If we try to apply brain organization theory to cultures further removed in time, these problems become even more obvious. A 1999 book
on homosexuality in ancient Roman culture begins: "Ancient Romans
lived in a cultural environment in which married men could enjoy sexual
relations with their male slaves without fear of criticism from their peers;
in which adultery generally aroused more concern than pederasty; in
which men notorious for their womanizing might be called effeminate,
while a man whose masculinity had been impugned could cite as proof
of his manhood the fact that he had engaged in sexual relations with his
accuser's sons."[19] How might prenatal androgen exposure account for all
that? Did Romans have endocrinological systems completely different
from ours?

Returning to the present day, we should note that the understanding
of sexual orientation and gender that is predominant among contemporary LGBT activists is that gender and sexual orientation form separate
and independent axes of identity (see illustration). For brain organization theory to support this claim, two separate causal mechanisms would
have to be found in the endocrine system, one for gender identity and

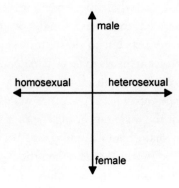

another for sexual orientation. To my knowledge, no one has proposed even the vaguest outlines of such a model, much less found any evidence for its existence. This has not stopped anyone who fervently believes that gender identity and sexual orientation are separate and independent from also believing that science has shown we are "born that way."

Nothing

At the end of the day, after Jordan-Young corrected for asymmetry and contradiction in the three hundred papers that constituted the entire field of brain organization theory up to the year 2000, what did she find?
    Nothing.
    All that research and writing and money and time over all those years, all the measuring and counting and coding, all the mutilated animals and surveillance of children's play, all the questionnaires and penile plethysmographs—all of it has yielded nothing that would count as scientific knowledge.
    The only conclusion that is consistently reported across symmetrical studies is that girls with classic CAH are more likely to play with "male" toys like cars and trucks than other girls. And they might also have slightly boyish playmate preferences and occupational interests, though this data is less clear.[20] Yet the research cannot distinguish whether this negligible effect is the result of prenatal events or the unique social experiences of girls with this rare disorder.
    Oh, and one more thing: symmetrical studies consistently reported that women with CAH are no more likely to be homosexual than other women.

When These Contradictions Become Political

The flaws of brain organization theory have direct political consequences, because the beliefs of the scientists are embraced by such a large number of LGBT activists and leaders. Thus the contradictions spill out of the laboratory and into the political arena. Let's look at one example in detail.
    In July 2010, Northwestern University issued a press release titled "Clinicians Attempt to Prenatally Prevent Homosexuality: Northwest-

ern Professor Protests Unapproved Use of Drug on Uninformed Patients." The release announced that Alice Dreger, a professor of bioethics at Northwestern's medical school, and her colleague Ellen Feder, a philosophy professor at American University, had "brought to national attention the first systematic approach to prenatally preventing homosexuality and bisexuality." Highlighting the gravity of the case, Dreger noted, "This is the first we know in the history of medicine that clinicians are actively trying to prevent homosexuality." At the same time, Dreger, Feder, and Anne Tamar-Mattis—an attorney and the director of Advocates for Informed Choice—published a piece on the *Bioethics Forum* website titled "Preventing Homosexuality (and Uppity Women) in the Womb?"[21]

Headlines in the major media followed, including "The Anti-Lesbian Drug," "Medical Treatment Carries Possible Side Effect of Limiting Homosexuality," and "Tempest in a Womb: What's Wrong with Preventing (or Promoting) Homosexuality in Utero?"[22] The reaction from LGBT rights organizations, activists, and scholars was immediate and outraged. Comparisons with the discredited eugenics practices of the early twentieth century were made.

At the center of the storm, once again, were girls with classic CAH.

Parental genetic testing can now determine which pregnancies are at risk for the disorder. And there is a drug, dexamethasone (DEX). If a woman who gives birth to a baby girl with classic CAH has taken DEX during pregnancy, the chances are good that the child's genitals will be typically female in appearance. This is a big deal. Parents of girls born with male-appearing genitalia often experience such profound anguish that they opt for surgeries to make their infant's genitalia appear more typically female. These surgeries, usually performed while the child is still an infant, are expensive, painful, often unsatisfactory, and can require serial corrective surgeries later on. All of that can now be avoided if the mother takes a little DEX pill while pregnant.

But there are downsides. DEX treatment must begin early in pregnancy, at a time when the odds are only one in eight that the fetus will actually become a girl with classic CAH. So for every one child who derives benefit from the treatment, seven will be needlessly exposed to the side effects of the drug. Those side effects are largely unknown and they will almost certainly remain so, since as we learned from our previous discussion of the DES controversy, the effects of exogenous chemicals that alter the prenatal hormonal milieu are extremely complex, take a wide variety of forms, and may not appear until late in the lives of offspring or even the offspring of offspring. Since classic CAH is a relatively rare disease that is not always prenatally diagnosed, and not every expectant mother who is diagnosed opts for DEX treatment, there are simply not enough cases to create the sample size that would be required for meaningful research. Studies of DEX treatment in rodents and primates suggest complications including low placental weight, low birth weight, small head circumference, cleft palate, adrenal hypoplasia, thymic hypoplasia, hepatomegaly, late-onset hypertension, and impaired glucose tolerance. But here we are right back at the debate about how much of what can be learned from rodents and primates applies to humans. There have been human cases that have indicated fetal growth retardation, and speculation that adverse outcomes would manifest primarily after middle age.[23]

In other words, it's a mess.

It will come as no surprise that the whole matter of prenatal DEX treatment has divided doctors, parents, and even adult women with CAH. This debate is now a decade old. Both sides have collected all the supporting documentation that can be mustered and made their case. People still disagree. Profoundly. On top of the stress of knowing she may give birth to a baby girl with a penis, a woman whose pregnancy has been diagnosed as at risk for classic CAH will receive passionate, even shrill, advice from all sides. Take the pill! Opt for surgery! Or just maybe: be a loving parent to a child with atypical genitalia who could have a harder time than most making her way in the world.

This would be a good time to note that there are other cultures which have accepted social roles for intersex individuals, so there is no need for surgery or pills, or even all that much anguish.[24]

Dr. Maria New is a particularly high-profile advocate of taking the pill. She is a professor of pediatrics and of genetics, as well as the director of the Adrenal Steroid Disorders Program, at the Mount Sinai School of Medicine. For almost forty years she was the director of Cornell University's Children's Clinical Research Center, and she served a term as president of the Endocrine Society. To make her case for prenatal DEX treatment even more persuasive to expectant mothers, she had been pitching an additional incentive: New explains to each of her patients that if she takes the pill, not only will her soon-to-arrive daughter have more typically female genitals, she will also be heterosexual.[25] She has repeated the claim both in her published papers and in lectures.[26]

New presented the research with which she supports this claim in a paper she published with Heino Meyer-Bahlburg, a psychologist who teaches at the Columbia University Medical Center, and two colleagues. Meyer-Bahlburg is one of the shining lights of brain organization theory and has published four decades of papers reporting on his search for a link between prenatal hormones and homosexuality. Titled "Sexual Orientation in Women with Classical or Non-classical Congenital Adrenal Hyperplasia as a Function of Degree of Prenatal Androgen Excess," the paper was published in 2008, around the same time New began speaking publicly about the ability of DEX to reduce homosexuality in women with CAH.[27] The paper prominently features many of the same methodological problems that plague the entire field of brain organization theory.

Early on in the paper, New and Meyer-Bahlburg admit that "early attempts to identify sex hormone abnormalities in human homosexuality were unsuccessful in men and only partially successful in women." This is already odd. Are New and Meyer-Bahlburg engaging in scientific research? If they are, then results demonstrating no relationship between sex hormone abnormalities and homosexuality would be just as "successful" as results showing the opposite. Or are they engaged in a sort of lab-based advocacy work, in which case their research is only "successful" if it produces an outcome that supports the positions they have advocated in debates such as whether pregnant women at risk for a CAH pregnancy should take DEX?

They follow with a review of studies that attempted to detect increased rates of homosexuality among CAH women, many of which were conducted by Meyer-Bahlburg himself. But these also fail to demonstrate the causal link they are searching for, leading New and Meyer-Bahlburg to conclude, "Clearly, more direct evidence of prenatal sex hormone effects would be desirable." Desirable? For what? In scientific research, results are considered desirable if they are accurate.

Meyer-Bahlburg and New hoped the new study would improve on these "undesirable" research outcomes by using a more fine-toothed comb to search for homosexuality among their research subjects. Perhaps previous studies failed to find a link between CAH and homosexuality because the search for homosexuality was not sufficiently diligent. They note that "many studies limited their data to the gender of actual sex partners or provided only quite limited detail on imagery." Perhaps if they dig down deeper into the personal lives of adults with CAH, heretofore hidden homosexuality will be discovered.

Thus women with CAH were queried about "masturbation fantasies, masturbation erotica, romantic/erotic fantasies during sexual relations with a partner, romantic/sexual daydreams, romantic/sexual night-dreams, sexual attractions, 'Total Imagery' [a composite of the preceding variables and the frequency of occurrence for each], and overall sexual responsiveness." Subjects were asked how often over their entire lifetime they had these fantasies, daydreams, and nightmares. All the answers were then indexed and coded into algorithms that yielded numbers which were placed on a scale of zero (heterosexual) to six (homosexual). When, at the end of the entire process, a number from zero to six had been assigned for each habit, daydream, hobby, or experience, the numbers were averaged down to one single number for each research subject. The zeros and ones were declared "heterosexual," while the twos, threes, fours, fives, and sixes were declared "bisexual" or "homosexual."

Again, CAH is an exceedingly rare disease, and not everyone wants to talk about this sort of thing with clinical researchers. Thus Meyer-Bahlburg and New were only able to round up sixty-one research subjects who have the type of CAH that results in atypical genitalia at birth, eighty-two with late-onset CAH that only becomes apparent later in life, and a control group of just twenty-four sisters and female cousins of the CAH group.

So what did they find? Women with CAH had more same-sex romantic and sexual partners than the control group. But as luck would have it, no one in the control group of twenty-four admitted to any same-sex romantic and sexual partners at all. In any such study, if the control value is zero, then even if just *one* woman with CAH had had just *one* same-sex liaison in her entire life, the study will have "found" a correlation between CAH and homosexuality in women. This is one of the problems of doing statistical research on tiny numbers of research subjects.

Thus, for the study to show a correlation between CAH and homosexuality in women, the data must come from some measure other than sexual partners: "masturbation fantasies, masturbation erotica, roman-tic/erotic fantasies during sexual relations with a partner, romantic/sex-ual daydreams, romantic/sexual nightdreams, sexual attractions, 'Total Imagery,'" and so on.

Of course, doctors are free to define whatever variables they wish in their research, but if they are going to present that research to the pub-lic as revealing some truth about homosexuality, then the definition of homosexuality used in their research must bear some resemblance to the way in which homosexuality is understood in the broader culture. When New and Meyer-Bahlburg criticize prior studies for "limiting their data to the gender of actual sex partners," they are very specifically criticizing those researchers for limiting their data to the "data" that is used by almost everyone else in the culture to determine who is homo-sexual and who is not. I suspect that there will be quite a few readers surprised to learn that New and Meyer-Bahlburg have diagnosed them as homosexual despite only having had sexual relations with opposite-sex partners for their entire lives.

One problem with the set of (always evolving) research procedures collectively known as "scientific method" is that they don't tell you when to stop—when to give up one line of research and pursue another. Mey-er-Bahlburg had been trying to find a causal relation between prenatal hormones and homosexuality for nearly forty years without success. In-stead of changing his research objectives, he expanded his definition of homosexuality to include women with masculinized genitalia who have sex exclusively with men yet occasionally fantasize about being the man in a sexual situation. This is absurd.

Imagine that New had been going around telling women at risk for CAH pregnancies that by taking a pill which in seven out of eight cases would needlessly expose their babies to possibly serious risk, they would reduce the chances that, in the eighth case, their daughter might at one point in her life have a romantic daydream about another woman. Would anyone have been impressed?

Keep in mind that New's research subjects are people with female-type chromosomes, a uterus, and ovaries, but genitals that may appear more like a penis and testicles than a vagina.[28] Should we be surprised to discover that when they daydream they "see themselves as men" more often than other women? CAH is also associated with obesity, short stature, body odor, acne, and more. People with CAH have more experience than most with doctors poking around their private parts, surveilling their play when they are children, and pressing them to answer surveys about their masturbation fantasies. Many have had one or more genital surgeries. Is anyone surprised that those in the CAH group fantasize (slightly) outside the box? What sort of research methodology would claim the ability to distinguish the consequences of having an atypical prenatal hormone milieu on one hand, and having the atypical experience of living with a highly medicalized body and mind on the other?

This research assumes that there are two human sexes (male and female), then asks whether prenatal hormone exposure determines which of three possible human sexual orientations these males and females eventually exhibit (heterosexual, homosexual, and bisexual). But these research subjects do not easily fit in the male or female boxes. In fact, one member of the research cohort was dropped from the study after deciding to switch from living as a woman to living as a man. A second subject was dropped for merely considering the same option. Meyer-Bahlburg and New cite the expulsion of these two subjects as evidence of the rigor of their research, but in fact it calls into question their most basic assumptions. If the boundary between male and female is unclear, then categories like homosexual (requiring two females or two males) are meaningless. When someone with female-type chromosomes, female-type breasts, and male-appearing genitals has sex with a woman, who is to say if that is "homosexual"? If it is, and the same person switches to living as a man and has sex with a woman, is that now "heterosexual"? This problem is fundamental, and cannot be solved by expelling from the study those who refuse to live by the researchers' assumptions.

Even beyond all of that, there is a punch line. Remember that Jordan-Young showed that only one logical conclusion could be drawn from a symmetry analysis of all the three-hundred-plus papers published in the entire field over four decades: that there is no correlation between CAH and homosexuality in women. Meyer-Bahlburg and New hoped that their absurd hunt for hidden homosexuality in the imaginations of their research subjects would prove a correlation between CAH and homosexuality in women. Yet the only thing that all the research in their field had clearly established was that no such correlation exists.

Stephen Jay Gould and the Mismeasure of Gender

There is not much the whole morass of brain organization theory can tell us about human sexual behavior, but there is a lot we can learn from it about the methods and pitfalls of scientific research. Thus it will be worth our while to take a brief detour from our historical narrative to consider how the work of a particularly deep thinker about scientific method might bear on the debacle of brain organization theory.

Stephen Jay Gould's magisterial *The Mismeasure of Man,* first published in 1981, is widely celebrated for debunking the large body of research that claimed to give scientific basis to the belief that some human races are more intelligent than others, and the corollary belief that the racial hierarchies of the contemporary world are a reflection of these measurable differences in intelligence. His specific targets were nineteenth-century craniometry (the measurement of skull volume and its relation to intelligence) and twentieth-century IQ measurement through psychological testing. More broadly, Gould took on what he called "the myth that science itself is an objective enterprise." In so doing, he presaged much of the work that has dominated the humanities ever since, and *The Mismeasure of Man* is considered a classic of late twentieth-century scholarship.[29]

In the introduction to an expanded edition published fifteen years later, Gould notes that "*The Mismeasure of Man* treats one particular form of quantified claim about the ranking of human groups: the argument that intelligence can be meaningfully abstracted as a single number capable of ranking all people on a linear scale. . . . This limited subject embodies the deepest (and most common) philosophical error, with the most fundamental and far-ranging social impact, for the entire troubling subject of nature and nurture."[30]

Early in the book Gould explains that this particular philosophical error rests on two "deep fallacies": the reification of complex sets of characteristics into a "unitary thing," and then measuring this "unitary thing" so as to rank individuals on a linear scale:

> The argument begins with one of the fallacies—*reification,* or our tendency to convert abstract concepts into entities (from the Latin *res,* or thing). We recognize the importance of mentality in our lives and wish to characterize it, in part so that we can make the divisions and distinc-

tions among people that our cultural and political systems dictate. We therefore give the word "intelligence" to this wondrously complex and multifaceted set of human capabilities. This shorthand symbol is then reified and intelligence achieves its dubious status as a unitary thing.

Once intelligence becomes an entity, standard procedures of science virtually dictate that a location and physical substrate be sought for it. Since the brain is the seat of mentality, intelligence must reside there.

We now encounter the second fallacy—*ranking,* or our propensity for ordering complex variation as a gradual ascending scale. . . .

But ranking requires a criterion for assigning all individuals to their proper status in the single series. And what better criterion than an objective number? Thus, the common style embodying both fallacies of thought has been quantification, or the measurement of intelligence as a single number for each person. This book, then, is about the abstraction of intelligence as a single entity, its location within the brain, its quantification as one number for each individual, and the use of these numbers to rank people in a single series.[31]

The Mismeasure of Man recounts in great detail how honest, highly trained men of science employed the most rigorous research procedures available to precisely measure brain sizes and psychological responses, yet achieved results that "recorded little more than social prejudice" and "invariably [found] that oppressed and disadvantaged groups—races, classes, or sexes—are innately inferior and deserve their status."[32]

Gould shows that once scientists begin from fallacious assumptions, measurement and theory become confounded, and even accurate measurement confirms instead of reveals the fallacies. He found this conflation of measurement and theory to be most prevalent in those sciences that date from the second half of the nineteenth century, when an "irresistible trend swept through the human sciences—the allure of numbers, the faith that rigorous measurement could guarantee irrefutable precision, and might mark the transition between subjective speculation and a true science as worthy as Newtonian physics."[33]

Gould pointed out that "the human body can be measured in a thousand ways," and that "any investigator, convinced beforehand of a group's inferiority, can select a small set of measures to illustrate its greater affinity with apes." Among his many examples was Etienne Serres, a nineteenth-century French anatomist who diligently and accurately measured the distance between navel and penis at various ages and found that "the navel migrates upward during growth, but attains greater heights in whites than in yellows, and never gets very far at all in blacks," and concluded that "blacks remain perpetually like white children and announce their inferiority thereby."[34]

Gould argued that these fallacies play out in a particularly vehement way when the subject of research is a touchy issue like race:

> Some topics are invested with enormous social importance but blessed with very little reliable information. When the ratio of data to social impact is so low, a history of scientific attitudes may be little more than an oblique record of social change. The history of scientific views on race, for example, serves as a mirror of social movements. This mirror reflects in good times and bad, in periods of belief in equality and in eras of rampant racism. The death knell of the old eugenics in America was sounded more by Hitler's particular use of once-favored arguments for sterilization and racial purification than by advances in genetic knowledge.[35]

How would it look if we were to apply Gould's critique of intelligence research to brain organization theory? All that is necessary is to substitute *gender* for *intelligence* in Gould's main argument. The critique would then be of the claim that "*gender* can be meaningfully abstracted as a single number capable of ranking all people on a linear scale," which, like claims about race, "embodies the deepest (and most common) philosophical error, with the most fundamental and far-ranging social impact, for the entire troubling subject of nature and nurture":

> We recognize the importance of *gender* in our lives and wish to characterize it, in part so that we can make the divisions and distinctions among people that our cultural and political systems dictate. We therefore give the word *"gender"* to this wondrously complex and multifaceted set of human capabilities. This shorthand symbol is then reified and *gender* achieves its dubious status as a unitary thing. Once *gender* becomes an entity, standard procedures of science virtually dictate that a location and physical substrate be sought for it. Since the brain is the seat of mentality, *gender* must reside there. We now encounter the second fallacy—ranking, or our propensity for ordering complex variation as a gradual ascending scale. . . .
>
> But ranking requires a criterion for assigning all individuals to their proper status in the single series. And what better criterion than an objective number? Thus, the common style embodying both fallacies of thought has been quantification, or the measurement of *gender* as a single number for each person. . . .

In a section titled "The Allure of Numbers," Gould makes some remarks about what he calls "'scientific' racism" that apply equally well to claims about gender and the validity of brain organization theory: "Science is rooted in creative interpretation. Numbers suggest, constrain, and refute; they do not, by themselves, specify the content of scientific theories. Theories are built upon the interpretation of numbers, and interpreters are often trapped by their own rhetoric. They believe in their own objectivity, and fail to discern the prejudice that leads them to one interpretation among many consistent with their numbers."[36]

8

The Contemporary Landscape

A century has passed since Eugen Steinach declared to the world in 1919 that "the question of the biological basis of homosexuality has been definitively solved."[1]

Fifty years later, Richard Green advised his colleague Robert Stoller, "Do not despair about the biological force behind gender identity. I am sure there is one somewhere."[2]

As I write these words, the "biological force behind gender identity" remains as obscure as ever, yet the clinical practices for medically treating gender "disorders," which were built on the belief that this biological force had been identified, have dramatically expanded and are now practiced on a global scale. None of the debates that erupted around these practices when they were located in the former animal house of Vienna's amusement park, or later in a handful of prestigious university hospitals, has been resolved, but the meeting point of gender identity and medical technology has shifted to a far less regulated social terrain where those debates are increasingly irrelevant.

Many of the forces at work in this shift are the same forces we encountered earlier when we watched testosterone escape the confines of traditional medical authority and wash over the nation as both cultural phenomenon and prized consumer item. The time is long past when a group of specialists can sit in conference room in the remote reaches of a university hospital and decide who can modify their body with hormones and surgery and who cannot. As with so many technologies, the two big forces at play are globalization and privatization.

The Globalization of Male-to-Female Technologies

In the United States, hormones for gender "transitioning" can be obtained at private clinics and some city-run clinics according to an "informed consent" model. All that is required is that the patient be able to document persistent "gender dysphoria" symptoms, demonstrate the "capacity to make a fully informed decision and to consent for treatment," and be at least twenty-one years of age; and that "if significant medical or mental health concerns are present, they must be reasonably well-controlled." And, of course, someone has to pay for it: either the patient, some form of insurance, or some form of public assistance. These criteria were first used in the early 1990s in San Francisco, conceived as a "harm reduction" approach that would give access to professional medical care to the many people in the city who were taking "street" hormones under no medical care at all. The criteria have since become an international norm, and in July 2012 were adopted into the seventh edition of the standards of care of the World Professional Association of Transgender Health (formerly the Harry Benjamin International Gender Dysphoria Association).[3]

Access to "top surgery" (surgical removal of breasts for female-to-males, surgical construction of female-appearing breasts for male-to-females) is available according to those same criteria. As surgery is far more expensive than hormone treatments, who pays for the surgery is a much bigger deal than who pays for hormones. Genital surgery usually requires a prior year on hormones living in one's preferred gender role. And even more money.

Gender technologies are subject to the same market pressures as automobiles and sneakers, so the production of gender "transition" has gone global like everything else. More sex reassignment surgeries are done in Thailand than anywhere else in the world. No one keeps a tally of exactly how many surgeries are done per year, but one prominent Thai surgeon who performs about two hundred surgeries a year himself estimated a national total of something like fifteen hundred a year in 2006. And the number has surely gone up since.[4]

People go to Thailand for surgery for the same reason that iPhones are manufactured in China. In Thailand, about US$8,000 buys a penile skin inversion vagina, which involves creating a cavity lined with skin from the penis. Those with more cash can opt for a colon vaginoplasty, in which a piece of the large intestine is used for the vaginal wall instead of the skin of the penis. The vascularized colon tissue can carry a blood supply and heal scar tissue if the new vagina collapses after the first surgery (subsequent corrective surgeries are still a regular occurrence for many gender transition procedures). Since the large intestine is bigger than the penis there is more tissue to work with, so the constructed cavity is more likely to be deep enough to be penetrated by a penis. In the United States, the same penile skin inversion will run approximately $12,000, and the colon vaginoplasty $26,000.

There is now a large menu of surgical procedures available to male-to-females. In addition to the removal of the penis and testicles and the construction of a vaginal cavity, one can add breast implants using any of a wide variety of techniques, a tracheal shave (to reduce the size of the Adam's apple), a scalp advance (to move the hairline down the forehead to a more typically female location), a reshaping of the forehead to a more feminine contour (lucky patients will have bone thick enough to be simply ground down, while others will have to have their foreheads essentially crushed and reconstructed), a brow lift (female eyebrows are typically higher than male), rhinoplasty (to give the nose a more feminine contour), cheek implants, lip lifts, lip filling, chin recontouring (again, grinding down the bone), jaw recontouring, vocal cord surgery (to raise the voice to a female pitch—testosterone will lower the pitch of a female voice, but estrogen will not raise the pitch of a male voice), and hand feminization surgery (to recontour the hand to more feminine proportions, by either grinding the bones or crushing and then reconstructing them). In the United States, the entire package can cost $200,000 or more. Thus the exodus of Americans to Thailand.

After Thailand, the country hosting the most sex reassignment surgery is Iran, where hormones and sex reassignment surgeries are fully paid for by a state that imposes the death penalty for homosexuality, in some cases by stoning. Ayatollah Ruhollah Khomeini, the spiritual Supreme Leader of Iran's 1979 Islamist revolution, issued a *fatwah* (religious edict) decreeing that homosexuals who submit to sex reassignment surgery and take partners of the opposite sex from the gender to which they have "transitioned" are acceptable in the eyes of Allah. Khomeini's ruling has an eerie similarity to Christine Jorgensen's more personal declaration: "I identified myself as female and consequently my interests in men were normal."[5]

As Hojatol-Islam Muhammad Mehdi Kariminiya, a Muslim cleric who is Iran's current leading expert on transgender theology, puts it: "Islam has a cure for people suffering from this problem. If they want to change their gender, the path is open. They need surgery. They are allowed to become either a male or a female. This discussion is fundamentally separate from a discussion regarding homosexuals. Absolutely not related. Homosexuals are doing something unnatural and against religion: they accept themselves."[6]

One of Iran's leading sex change surgeons explains how he discerns homosexuals from the transgendered: "A homosexual is never willing to operate. The first thing I do when I meet a patient is tell them that this operation is from hell. I tell them its an inhumane operation. You are going to be ripped apart. I give such a difficult and terrible description that a homosexual runs out of here by the third sentence. He says, 'That's not me.' A transexual says, 'That's my deep desire.'"

Note that what is being put into practice in Iran is Harry Benjamin's proposal that the request for surgery be used as the diagnostic criterion for the disease the surgery allegedly cures. Note also the similarities with John Money's "skyscraper test" for diagnosing homosexuality, though Money's threat of pushing the homosexual off a skyscraper was merely metaphorical. How the Iranian surgeon discerns the difference between actually wanting one's penis and testicles surgically removed, as opposed to wanting to avoid death by stoning, is left unexplained.

What do post-op male-to-females do in a conservative society under an Islamist regime? Many become Islam-approved prostitutes. As one such person explains: "We sell ourselves. We have certain principles. Whenever we are working, we first do a temporary Islamic marriage contract. It's allowed by Islam. Since we don't have female reproductive parts and cannot get pregnant, we can get married once an hour or so."

Globalization has taken the paradox that played out in the first half of the twentieth century within the confines of Europe and the United States and distributed it across the globe. Before globalization, men identified as homosexuals by police and medical authorities sometimes had estrogen and surgery forced on them against their will, while access to those same technologies was denied to men who requested it because of their wish to become women. Today, westerners with the necessary cash can travel to Thailand for all the "transitioning" money can buy, while Iranians can avoid the capital punishment meted out to homosexuals by opting instead for surgery and hormones.

The New Transmen

Female-to-male technology has taken a very different course. Early attempts at the surgical construction of penises produced unsatisfying and sometimes horrific results, and despite decades of effort surgeons remain unable to construct anything close to a penis in size, appearance, function, or sensation. The techniques available leave visible scarring from skin grafts taken from elsewhere on the body, can involve multiple surgeries, and are expensive, painful, slow to heal, and fraught with complications.

In recent years an increasing number of female-to-males have opted to skip genital surgery altogether and settle for double mastectomies ("top surgery") and testosterone-based pharmaceutical products that stimulate growth of facial hair and muscle mass, redistribute body fat, and lower the voice. This mix of procedures alters the patient's public or clothed appearance in ways that read socially as male, while avoiding the pain, cost, and disappointing outcomes of penis construction surgery. The genitals, however, do not remain unchanged. Testosterone causes the clitoris to grow noticeably larger and also gives it new function. Transmen today speak of their newly acquired ability to "get a hard on" and of a range of pleasurable and previously unknown sensations available from their enlarged clitorises, which complement what they report to be a dramatically elevated sexual desire.[7] It was from this combination of top surgery and hormones that both the *transman* as an individual and *transgender* as an identity emerged, shifting the designation of *transexual* to those who opt for genital surgery as well.

When the reconfigured transman appeared, the effect was literally electric, as transman images were circulated on the Internet, itself a new phenomenon at the time. One transman doctor who was going through school at the time remembers his experience like this:

> I got immensely frustrated because I would read [medical journals that] would show pictures of these phalloplasties [surgically constructed pe-

nises]. . . . "Oh my God, this isn't what I want. This is crazy, I'm not doing this." . . . In college, I similarly had access to medical literature, and I said, "I'm never doing that." When I was in medical school, I was like, "Whoa, now I got some really good access to stuff," and I knew how to research the medical literature, and yet . . . I was never gonna transition because it just wasn't good enough. When I went to residency, same thing.

Then in 2002 I didn't have ready access to a medical library but I did have the Internet, so I said, "Well why don't we do a little research here?" And for the first time, I saw descriptions and pictures of [transmen]. I spent two or three hours on the Internet, I realized what was possible, and I said, "I'm doing this right now." In medical [journals] they talk about people's functionality and they show pictures of phalloplasties, but they don't show you pictures of transmen. If they show you a face, they got the eyes blocked out. It looks pretty sad. But when you put a face on it. . . . Within a week or two, I actually met the first transman I ever met, and he was just a dude, like indistinguishable from any other guy I'd ever seen. And I was like, "Oh my God I have to do this. This is what I am."[8]

The appearance of large numbers of transmen in urban sexual subcultures marked a sea change in queer culture. Beginning with the earliest medical treatises on gender-variant behavior in the late nineteenth century and continuing for one hundred years, both medical authorities and campaigners for the rights of sexual minorities assumed that male-to-females far outnumbered female-to-males, and sometimes even debated whether female-to-males existed at all. With the emergence of the transman the tables turned. Particularly in New York City and San Francisco, where the political weight of the LGBT community has resulted in easier access to hormones and top surgery than elsewhere in the country, transmen suddenly seemed to be everywhere. One young person in her late twenties who had been debating whether to "transition" recounted how, over the course of one year, she noted the presence of more transmen on each visit she made to San Francisco's most prominent lesbian bar. "The other day," she recounted, "I realized that if I want to hang out with butch dykes, I have to hang out with people older than me, because among my friends all the butch dykes have become transmen."[9]

Many new transmen identified themselves as lesbians before going on pharmaceuticals. They had been active in lesbian social and political networks, and they do not view their engagement with these technologies as placing themselves outside of the communities in which they had made their lives. Many have partners who consider themselves lesbians and have also made their lives in lesbian culture. In contrast, there is a well-established though extremely discreet subculture of men who are sexually attracted to transwomen, but these men rarely think of themselves as gay and often go to great lengths to avoid contact with the gay social world.

This contrasts sharply with previous generations whose tenor was set by prominent male-to-female transexuals like Christine Jorgensen, who not only rejected gay identity prior to transition but was publicly and explicitly homophobic. Jorgensen's declaration that homosexuality was "deeply alien to my religious attitudes" even prompted one of her admirers to write to her suggesting that she become a missionary devoted to saving homosexuals from sin (a role for which she would have received state support in contemporary Iran).[10] Or Virginia Prince, who coined the word *transgender* and explicitly forbid homosexuals (whom she regarded as "emotionally disturbed people") from joining the first transgender organization, which she founded. Jorgensen and Prince would have been as appalled at homosexuals seeking to publicly align themselves with early transpeople as the current transgender generation is appalled when today's gay and lesbian community try to shut them out. Many transgender people of today very much want to be included in the queer umbrella, and, as we've seen, it is their activism that has added the T to LGBT.

Gender Transition, Gender Enhancement

Paradoxically, the increasingly urgent insistence that "T" belongs with LGB comes at the same time that the act of reconstructing one's gender with hormones and ancillary technologies has experienced explosive growth in mainstream culture. Almost every item on the menu of technologies available for "transitioning" from male to female is also employed by women-born-women, and in far greater numbers: rhinoplasties, cheek implants, lip lifts, lip fillings, chin recontouring, jaw recontouring, and more. The same techniques that are considered *gender transition* technologies when performed on someone born male are considered *rejuvenation* technologies when performed on someone born female. In other words, the woman that male-to-females want to become is a woman that women-born-women cannot become without employing the very same technologies. It is an embodiment of "womanhood" that must be technologically constructed, no matter what body you start out with.

One of the reasons there are fewer entries on the menu of technologies for the female-to-male is that the market among straight men for "male rejuvenation" technologies has been far smaller than the market among straight women for "female rejuvenation," but this is changing rapidly with the rise of highly profitable male rejuvenation clinics cashing in on the popularity of testosterone. Go to almost any urban gym, gay or straight, and you will see male bodies amped up on testosterone. Straight men can each now spend $60,000 and more on "rejuvenation," paying more to construct an amplified male gender than most female-to-males spend on "transitioning."[11] Here again, the male body everyone wants is a body that very few can have without hormone technologies, no matter what body they were born into. Whether referred to as "gender transition" for transmen, "rejuvenation" for straight men, or "sports doping" for athletes, the technology is the same.

The debate about which men-born-men should have access to these technologies is a long and convoluted one, with many parallels to the debate about transgender access to the same. It is no closer to being resolved today than it ever was, but just as in the world of "gender transition," the privatization and globalization of medicine has made the technologies used for male rejuvenation and sports doping so readily available that the debate about who should have access is fading into irrelevance.

The John Money of the sports doping world was Dr. Robert Kerr, who in the 1970s and 1980s spoke openly and passionately about administering hormones to several thousand athletes, body-builders, and policemen, and published a sort of doping manifesto in 1982 that attempted to establish athletic hormone enhancement as standard medical practice. Like many transgender health-care providers, Kerr saw his athletic hormone practice not in terms of building more competitive athletes, but rather as a form of harm reduction and confirming sense of self: "Body building has taken literally thousands of short, small and shy men out of their doldrums and produced a new generation of well-built men with a sound sense of pride and self-confidence. . . . Athletes are going to take anabolic steroids. But the vast majority of athletes in this country are not taking drugs under anyone's supervision."[12]

Dr. Kerr later dropped his athletic hormone practice, explaining that his attempt at harm reduction had failed because his patients so often supplemented what he prescribed with drugs they obtained elsewhere. Kerr's experience foreshadowed that of a doctor interviewed for this book, who left his job at San Francisco's city clinic for transgender care in part as a result of frustration over how many of his transgender patients were supplementing the hormones supplied free by the city with higher doses purchased on the street. They did this in the hope that it would accelerate their "transition," but all it did was increase their health risks.[13]

"Puberty to Grave"

Children are being swept up in the hormone wave at younger and younger ages. Even high school athletes are doping. But the youngest Americans receiving "sex hormone" medicine are children diagnosed with Gender Dysphoria and given "hormone blockers," pharmaceutical products that inhibit the body's production of androgens and estrogens and thus delay the onset of puberty. The rationale is that although preteen children are too young to make the decision to "transition" to another gender, if they were to begin gender transition hormone therapy before adolescence their appearance would be more convincing in their new gender. So instead of beginning hormone therapy immediately, they are put on medication that shuts down the metabolic processes of adolescence, and will thus arrive at an age that is considered old enough to make an informed decision on hormone treatment with a pre-adolescent body.

The use of hormone blockers in children was initiated by Dr. Norman Spack, founder of the Gender Management Service at Boston Children's Hospital in 2008. Similar clinics now exist in San Francisco, Los Angeles, Chicago, Denver, Minneapolis, New York, Hartford, Providence, and Washington, DC. In almost all of these places there is a doctor Spack has trained or mentored.

Spack is supremely confident that he can reliably diagnose "gender dysphoria" in children, and reliably distinguish between homosexual and transgender children. "Gender dysphoria is a condition that can be treated rather easily," he says. "You don't need to be a rocket scientist." He has two diagnostic criteria: The child must exhibit a "strong and persistent desire" to change gender; and must be in ongoing mental health counseling. That's it. To begin therapy, consent from both parents is also required.

Kyle Smith is one nine-year-old who met Spack's criteria. Kyle was so convinced of his own diagnosis that right there in the doctor's office he turned to his father and said, "Dad, I need help. You need to help me. You need to tell Dr. Spack. I need medical help." Kyle later told a journalist that he remembered looking at Spack as "some kind of god."[14]

Given that doctors, scholars, and transgender activists have been unable to agree on which *adults* are transgender and which are not, why such confidence in distinguishing transgender *nine-year-olds*? Over the last decade, debates among transgender adults about who is and is not transgender have only become deeper and more bitter. What tone will these debates take in ten or twenty years, when the voices of those whose parents and doctors put them on hormone blockers at age nine are added to the mix?

Steroid hormones are the only medication that have an effect on every cell and organ in the body. Many of these effects have not been sufficiently studied. For example, we now know that the hormones that flow through adolescents at puberty trigger growth not just of facial hair and breasts but also of the brain, which undergoes a significant but poorly understood transformation as a result.[15] Children given hormone blockers to prevent the growth of breasts or hair might not grow a third arm, but will they miss out on brain growth that would have otherwise occurred?

Imagine the scale of study that would be required to develop anything close to a complete understanding of the consequences of preventing adolescence in a child. The Women's Health Initiative had 160,000 subjects and yielded inconclusive results. Should we round up 160,000 kids? Who would be followed throughout their entire lives? Continually tested for brain function and every sort of behavior? There will never be such a study, beginning with the fact that there will likely never be 160,000 such kids.

With the administration of hormone blockers to preadolescents at the beginning of life and the administration of estrogen and testosterone to elderly women and men at the end of life, William H. Masters's call for "puberty to grave sex steroid support" has become an American reality. If we consider fetal exposure to endocrine disrupting chemicals, the trajectory is extended from womb to grave.

Conclusion

In the summer of 2013, Private First Class Bradley Manning was sentenced to thirty-five years in a maximum-security prison at Fort Leavenworth for leaking classified US military documents relating to the Iraq war to WikiLeaks. The next day Manning announced through a spokesperson that she would henceforth identify herself as Chelsea Manning and asked "to begin hormone therapy as soon as possible." Lauren McNamara, a transgender activist who became an online confidante of Manning in 2009 and later was the only transperson to testify for the defense at Manning's court-martial hearing, spoke to the media to explain and support Manning's request for hormone therapy: "There is not another side of this from a scientific or medical perspective. There is not dissent here. There is not a debate here. And anyone who acts as though this is not legitimate, as if this is not real, as if this is not a medical necessity, is simply uninformed and should not have a place in any discussion over this."[1]

As a queer, a pacifist, a donor to Manning's defense fund, and person who thinks all people should have the right to do with their bodies as they please, I fully support Chelsea Manning's right to do with her body as she pleases. But by McNamara's criteria, the history presented in this book should not be published, or "have a place in any discussion over this." But one could not stop with this book. Debate and dissent concerning the source of gender and sexual variance—whether these have a single source in the body that can be quantified and measured, whether they constitute a disease, and whether hormones are an appropriate treatment—these debates have been so central to queer history for over a hundred years that pretending this is not the case would require hiding away or rewriting huge chunks of that history.

Just a few years before the Manning trial, San Francisco's famed LGBT film festival canceled a movie it had programmed when trans activists protested that the film was transphobic. This marked the first time since the festival began in 1977 that a film had been censored. The film was a very low-budget short by a longtime lesbian filmmaker, Catherine Crouch, whose numerous other films had showed in many queer film festivals over the years without problem. It portrayed a 1970s lesbian knocking her head during a volleyball game and waking up decades later in a dystopian future in which men were allowed to have sex with men, and women with women, as long as one partner changed genders beforehand. It was a comedy. A humorous, sci-fi take on Iran as played out in, say, New Jersey. A community forum was called to discuss the festival's decision to censor the movie. Susan Stryker, who had led the effort to cancel the film, declared that it deserved censorship because it "left too much room for misinterpretation." Yet this could be used as the very definition of art: something that leaves room for (mis) interpretation.

Free speech has long been a core value of the queer community. Before 1958, it was illegal for activists to discuss homosexuality in print.[2] Newspapers reported on police raids of queer bars by obliquely referring to "degenerates" or "men with a feminine bent."[3] The 1958 Supreme Court ruling which changed all that is the victory on which all other queer victories stand. How did we get from there to censoring movies in queer film festivals because they leave too much room for misinterpretation?

Two Identities

The idea of identity pervades queer culture to a degree unequaled anywhere else. But we use the term *identity* in two very different, even opposing ways. There is the identity in "identity politics," and there is the identity in "gender identity." We often slip back and forth between the two meanings without noticing. This creates all kinds of confusion, leakages, and feedbacks between the two.

The identity in "identity politics" refers to a shared experience of oppression, and perhaps to how that shared experience is manifest through shared social struggle.[4] It is a declaration of something many have in common. It is not something that can be "disordered" in one individual, and a person's identity in the "identity politics" sense cannot be made to "transition" from one thing to another with pharmaceutical products.

The identity in "gender identity" is something strictly individual. It is synonymous with "personality" and eventually blurs into "ego." It is an identity of one. It can be diagnosed by a medical professional as disordered, and treated with commercially produced pharmaceutical products.

This single word can thus refer to things as distinct as, say, the shared experiences of the Black feminist collective who are credited with coining the term "identity politics" on the one hand, and the relationship between a single individual's mind and body on the other. It can do both at the same time, and even flip back and forth between meanings without anyone noticing. Transgender activism is situated precisely at the point where the two meanings of identity meet, and thus can employ the word to marshal all the moral and political weight of shared oppression in the service of an individual ego. And since this identity is alleged to reside in hormone levels that can be pharmaceutically manipulated, the political and moral claims of identity expand to encompass all the relevant technologies.

Two Transphobias

The different meanings of identity have a mirror image in the different meanings of the word *transphobia*. Here again the word carries two very different meanings, and we slip back and forth between the two without noticing. This creates all kinds of confusion, leakages, and feedbacks between the two. It can mean an irrational fear of gender-variant behavior or appearance, in the same sense that "homophobia" refers to an irrational fear of same-sex eroticism. But *transphobia* is also applied to any expression of doubt that gender is something that can be modified with technology. By conflating social acceptance of certain *behaviors* or *sense of self* with agreement as to the *meaning of a specific set of technologies*, transphobia provides an easy checkmate against anyone who celebrates every sort of gender expression and behavior while remaining skeptical of whether chemical or surgical technologies can cause a person to "transition" from male to female or vice versa.

Two Histories

Transgender history, as it has been told in a number of general transgender histories and in an even larger number of personal narratives, is the history of an identity and those who so identify. It is very much a history of personal and social struggle: how people who classify themselves as transgender think and feel about themselves, their struggle to be seen in the same way by the broader culture, and who they find to be most like themselves when they look back through history.

At the center of this story is a history that now extends back a hundred years of people demanding that medical authorities give them access to "sex hormone" technologies, demands that were in nearly every case denied. In this narrative, the last ten years is a time of unprecedented victories. Years of struggle have finally cracked open the medicine chest. Thousands of people now receive hormones who in previous times would have been denied them, often through health insurance coverage for employees of large corporations, or health clinics in a few large cities that offer free hormones. These programs are the direct fruits of social struggle.

But what happens if we expand the historical subject to include everyone who has engaged with "sex hormone" technology: the beliefs people have held about "sex hormones," their struggle to get access to these technologies, and what happened when they acted on these beliefs? Viewed through this lens, the present day no longer seems so unique. There have been many times when what we call activism today has been successfully employed by people wanting to access "sex hormone" technologies. I will recall just two of many such cases. Concerns about the safety of the first synthetic estrogen kept approval of DES for use in women held up in the FDA until a wave of letters from women around the country demanding access to the drug poured into Congress and the White House. During the heyday of Battey's Operation, women went from doctor to doctor demanding to have their ovaries removed because they believed this would bring them relief from acute mental anguish. Doctors who refused were rebuked. If we were to put those rebukes into the vocabulary of present-day activism, these doctors were accused of misogyny.

DES and Battey's Operation are today considered two of the biggest catastrophes in the history of medicine. It took years for their tragedies to unravel. DES was approved for use in women for more than forty years. Millions of women took it. The doctors who prescribed it were supremely confident in its safety. When the scale of its negative effects finally came into view, it was not because women who had taken it went to doctors complaining of side effects; the effects were too far removed from the act of taking the pills for anyone to connect the two. Years had to pass. The women's daughters had to grow to adolescence in sufficient numbers for rare cancers to appear. Likewise, the end of Battey's Operation did not result from the complaints of women who underwent the surgery.

By the first definition of transphobia—an irrational fear of gender-variant behavior or appearance—there is nothing transphobic about this book. To the contrary, history is a tool for empowering and understanding. But if this book is judged according to the second definition—that any expression of doubt that gender is something that can be modified with technology is transphobic—we have problems, because the history told here casts doubt in all directions. By simply telling the story of all the medical tragedies and intellectual debacles that constitute the history of "sex hormones," we cannot avoid the suggestion that the medical practices we pursue today and the meaning we ascribe to them may someday fall from favor.

Thus, by the second meaning of transphobia, this history should simply not be told. Better to hide it away.

Let us consider three possible responses to the larger perspective we gain when we move from a transgender history to a history of "sex hormones." None of these responses is "right" or "wrong," but I will note a problem with each.

In the first case, we might thank our lucky stars that after all the confusion and heartbreak and tragedy of the last hundred years, we have the good fortune of living at the time when science is finally getting gender "right," and when years of activism have finally won access to the chemicals some queers urgently need.

The problem here is the assumption that every generation before us got things wrong and we are the first generation to get things right. This is a common fallacy with how we perceive history, no matter what history we consider. On what grounds do we assume that we have a more perfect self-awareness and self-knowledge than all our predecessors? Or that our technologies will be the first technologies in history that will not vex us with unintended consequences?

In the second case, we might acknowledge that the history casts doubt on present-day technologies, but we would add that there is nothing unique about the history of "sex hormone" medicine, that the entire history of medicine is full of similar tragedies and debacles, but that doesn't mean we should not make use of all the powerful technologies now available to us.

The problem with this second case is that it may not be true, and at the very least it is overstated. While it is true that there have been many cases in many fields in which medical procedures were revealed to cause more harm than good, the history of "sex hormone" medicine may be unique in its uninterrupted series of large-scale catastrophes. There are good reasons that this would be so. The idea that there are chemical essences of manhood and womanhood has repeatedly excited the imaginations of scientists, clinical doctors, journalists, patients, and capitalists in ways that other drugs and technologies have not. Over and over, this excitement has led all parties to throw caution to the wind, with disastrous consequences each time. Furthermore, the precise ways in which exogenous "sex hormones" affect the endocrine system and the rest of the body have proven to be remarkably hard to pin down. And this has in turn amplified the tendency to throw caution to the wind, since waiting for a more certain understanding of the mechanisms at play could mean waiting for a very long time indeed. Finally, "sex hormones" clearly have some sort of impact on human behavior, but measuring human behavior leads to problems for which scientific method has no ready answer. (I will have more to say about the "looping effect" of measuring human behavior shortly.)

In the third case, the take-away from our story would be a greater awareness about the limits of scientific knowledge based on measuring human behavior, less confidence in both the efficacy and safety of current technologies, and a greater awareness of the role that the hunt for profits has played in the spread of the belief that gender has a chemical essence. All in all, we would take away a greater humility about contemporary beliefs about gender, identity, biology, and technology, and an awareness that in all likelihood these too shall pass.

The problem here is that humility in our beliefs about technology is not an easy fit with transgender activism and medical practices. The idea that a pharmaceutical product can cause gender to transition, confidence that we can safely take drugs over a long period of time that affect the body's metabolic processes in very deep and poorly understood ways, confidence that we can safely shut down adolescence in children—these are hardly humble claims. To the contrary, they are audacious. That audacity was well expressed by Christine Jorgensen when, in the 1950s, she compared the technology she was using to transition from male to female to the technology that would soon put a man on the moon.[5]

Once a person has engaged such audacious technology to alter his or her body and sense of self in what he or she perceives to be irrevocable ways, it may be profoundly uncomfortable and even painful for that person to question the meaning of the technology, or to hear someone else do the same. This is reasonable and understandable. After having gone through extreme unhappiness, psychotherapy, medical screening, health insurance screening, family rejection, extended pharmaceutical treatment, and even extremely painful and invasive surgeries, the last thing anyone wants to hear is a questioning of those very technologies.

And yet question we must. We are living at a time of unprecedented technological change. New options to modify our bodies, from muscle mass to brain chemistry, are multiplying, as are the options for sharing our new appearance on Facebook and YouTube via those laptops and smartphones we cannot tear ourselves away from. Every new option for personal expression and identity brings with it new options for surveillance and control. Moving from the personal to the global, on every hand environmental crises threaten to overwhelm. I noted earlier that at the largest scale, we are living at a time when human technology is causing the earth's climate to warm, the seas to acidify, and—as a result of the rapid increase of industrial-scale production of endocrine disrupting chemicals—living tissue to become more estrogenic. Questioning the meanings and uses of technology is the most urgent task of our time.

Here we arrive back at where we began in the introduction to this book. I find it profoundly distressing that my community, the queer community, has developed a politics which asserts that there are certain

meanings of technology it is unacceptable to question. That once someone has used a given technology to alter their sense of self, any questioning of that technology is out of bounds.

Can we find a way to respect those whose sense of self is deeply entwined with particular beliefs about technology while at the same time
leaving those beliefs open to question? If we can do this, we will indeed
be making a contribution to a society in which many others will be confronting similar dilemmas in the near future. One measure of how well
we succeed will be how freely we can study our own history.

Who Is Sick?

Beyond the health risks involved in "sex hormone" medicine, queers
pay a high social and political price for interfacing so deeply with the
power structure of the medical industry. Whether that price is worth the
benefit the technologies provide is a question each person must answer
for him/her/their selves. But without seriously considering the cost, it is
impossible to answer the question at all.

In the very earliest days of homophile and homosexual activism in
the 1950s, activists debated whether those doctors and psychiatrists who
had the least horrible understanding of homosexuality could be of any
use to their nascent movement. But from the 1960s on, gay and lesbian
activists became remarkably unified in their assertion that *we are not
sick,* that *the only experts on lesbians and gays are lesbians and gays,* and
that *there is nothing doctors and psychiatrists have to offer us other than to
leave us alone.* At its core, this was the liberation in the "gay liberation"
movement of the late 1960s and 1970s, and what distinguished "gays and
lesbians" from those who declared themselves "homosexual": "homosexuals" remained open to the idea that they had a medical problem that
medical experts might help them with; "gays" were emphatic that they
had no problem other than society's intolerance. Thus the slogan "Gay
is Good." Just as feminists proclaimed that "taking control of our own
lives and of our bodies is the most basic feminist principle there is," gay
liberationists believed that taking control of their own lives and bodies
was the most basic principle of gay liberation.[6]

Note that at the time, the term *gay* functioned much like *queer* does
today: gays were male or female, with a range of gender expression from

mainstream to flamboyantly transgressive. What made you gay was your assertion that your same-sex attraction was a good thing, your desire to participate in the social upheavals of the era, and for many a belief that those outside the sexual mainstream had a unique perspective that could make a useful addition to those struggles. Many (though certainly not all) people who feel their mode of gender expression makes them trans today would have considered themselves gay during the gay liberation years.

Conversely, dealing with the medical power structure has been a life-long priority for transpeople from Lili Elbe to Christine Jorgensen to Reed Erickson to Susan Stryker. As the transgender identity took off in the mid-1990s and was embraced by ever larger numbers of people, more and more queers spent more and more of their lives dealing with doctors, psychiatrists, psychologists, surgeons, pharmacies, and insurance companies. Thus the rise of the transgender identity has swung the interface between queer people and medical authority strongly in the opposite direction it was headed in the 1960s and 1970s.

Hormones can only be legally obtained by prescription, and sex reassignment surgery is not something that activists can perform for themselves, so people who desire to engage with those technologies do indeed need experts and authorities. As a result, many trans activists have for decades insisted that *we are sick* and thus *we deserve medical help.* This thread has been cross-weaved with another, very different impulse that asserts there is nothing "sick" about being transgender, that transgender is an "embodied place that is technologically constructed" and is both empowering and subversive. But health insurance is reserved for people who are sick, and the mantle of an "embodied place that is technologically constructed"[7] can just as easily describe all the aging men and women using hormones and surgery to appear younger than their years, procedures deemed "cosmetic" and thus not covered by insurance. So the *we are not sick* position has always been embraced by a minority among transpeople, and the distance between the two positions accounts for much of the animosity that has been so prominent within the trans community.

In 1973, when homosexuality was *removed* from the American Psychiatric Association's *Diagnostic and Statistical Manual of Mental Disorders* (*DSM*) and no longer classified as a mental illness, it was the result of years of activism by lesbians and gays who passionately demanded its removal. In 1980, when Gender Identity Disorder was *added* to the *DSM,* it was likewise the culmination of years of activism by transpeople who just as passionately demanded its inclusion. Gays wanted *out* because they were adamant they were not sick. Trans activists wanted *in* because getting into the *DSM* is the key that unlocks health insurance. No diagnosis in the *DSM* = no money from health insurance.

This is not to say that all trans activists have been comfortable with being cornered into claiming an illness. Many are not. Thus, as the result of trans activism, the fifth edition of the *DSM,* published in 2013, reclassified transgender people as suffering from Gender Dysphoria instead of Gender Identity Disorder. And within the world of transgender medicine, the authorities considered the most open to the voices of trans activists now use the word *consumer* in place of *patient.*[8]

Words, however, cannot change the fact that hormone treatment is either covered by health insurance or it is not. And this will be determined by whether it is listed as a sickness in the *DSM* or it is not.

There is an intellectual current now formulating in academia and trans health care that is trying to articulate an argument that health insurance should cover hormones and surgery *and* that there is no transgender pathology. This was a big part of why the 2013 *DSM* changed the diagnosis from "Gender Identity Disorder" to "Gender Dysphoria." Maybe if you have a "dysphoria" instead of a "disorder" you can be pathology-free but still get health insurance. This is a word game. Gender Dysphoria is the only diagnosis in the *DSM* that uses the term.

Several transgender activists with whom I have discussed these issues responded by asserting that neither they nor any of their transgender friends actually believed they were sick; they just said that to get hormones—in their words, to "game the system." But who is gaming whom? The pharmaceutical industry is a multibillion-dollar beast with a great big megaphone.

It's not as if the stories about ourselves that we tell psychiatrists, doctors, and social workers exist in one world, and the stories about ourselves that we tell each other exist in another. We cannot keep them apart. The meanings of sexual identities emerge from the lives and practices and discourses of those identified. The present meaning of *transgender* emerged from a process in which doctors, psychiatrists, judges, cops, scholars, and other expert authorities have been ever more deeply entwined. And again, at the center of it all are pharmaceutical products sold by huge corporations at a profit. In the process, at least to some extent, what began as a movement for sexual liberation has become a movement for patient and consumer rights.

The change becomes most vivid if we focus our gaze on the treatment of children. In the 1970s and 1980s, many queers arrived in the gay enclaves of big cities with painful memories of childhoods in which they had endured a kind of torture at the hands of doctors and psychiatrists who treated their gender-variant behavior as a medical disease. Saving future generations from such painful experiences was at the top of their agenda: *Leave queer children alone! There is nothing wrong with them. They don't need doctors. What they need is a bus ticket to San Francisco and a warm welcome when they arrive. Yes, they are minors, but they are effectively being tortured, and they need to escape.*

Today, transgender activists agitate with the same fervor for access to hormone blockers for preadolescent queer kids. *Queer children need medical help! There is nothing wrong with giving it to them. Yes, they are minors, but their bodies are going through changes that demand immediate medical intervention.*

The idea that certain kinds of childhood gender experience require medical intervention is now so deeply ingrained in our culture that a nine-year-old can sit in the *Gender Management office* of Boston Children's Hospital and cry out, "Dad, I need help. You need to help me. You need to tell Dr. Spack. I need medical help."

Two Loops

From the birth of modern psychiatry and endocrinology, queers have been caught in what the philosopher Ian Hacking calls the "looping effect": how scientific classifications of people "affect the people classified, and how the effects on the people in turn change the classifications."[9]

Hacking notes that when a new scientific classification of a kind of person (homosexual or transgender, for example) is declared, as the people who fall within the new classification become aware of being classified, they will experience that classification as a "way to be a person." As a result of experiencing life in this new way, with this new identity, the classified people "enhance and adjust what is true of them," and the original classification must then be duly altered to account for the change, and another trip around the loop begins. Hacking argues that this loop gives sciences that classify humans by measuring their behavior a fundamentally different dynamic from other sciences, because their classifications are "moving targets." These sciences include "many social sciences, psychology, psychiatry, and a good deal of clinical medicine."[10]

Hacking argues that this dynamic is increasingly fundamental to how we understand ourselves and form ourselves as subjects: "Only in the past two hundred years have the sciences been so central to the human understanding of who we are. We make ourselves in our own scientific image of the kinds of people it is possible to be."[11]

To assess the relevance of this claim to the subject matter of this book, think back to Magnus Hirschfeld's Scientific-Humanitarian Committee, the first queer rights organization of the modern era, whose slogan was "Justice Through Science," and was housed in Hirschfeld's Institute for Sexual Science in Berlin. Remember how the race to isolate and then synthesize estrogen and testosterone laid the foundations of today's pharmaceutical industry, which continues to be dominated by the huge corporations that were the big winners in that original race. Remember how synthetic estrogen became one of the first prescription drugs and a model for all that followed. Remember how the dispute over estrogen marketing was the wedge that opened the door to direct-to-consumer drug marketing, and that "sex hormones" are some of the most profitable pharmaceutical products in history.

Hacking initially fleshed out the dynamic of his "looping effect" of scientific classifications of humans studying Dissociative Identity Disorder:

> Around 1970 there arose a few sensational paradigm cases of strange behaviour similar to phenomena discussed a century earlier and largely forgotten. A few psychiatrists began to diagnose multiple personality. It was rather sensational. More and more unhappy people started manifesting these symptoms. At first they had the symptoms they were expected to have. But then they became more and more bizarre. First a person had two or three personalities. Within a decade the mean number was seventeen. This fed back into the diagnoses, and entered the standard set of symptoms. It became part of the therapy to elicit more and more alters. . . . This became a way to be a person.[12]

Gender Identity Disorder and Dissociative Identity Disorder have a lot in common. They were the first—and to date the only—mental health diagnoses to incorporate the word *identity*, and they both made it into the *DSM* at the same time, in 1980. ("Dissociation" was first ushered into the modern world by Jean-Martin Charcot, a doctor who became a celebrity by having his female patients give stunning performances of "hysterical fits" for the nineteenth-century Parisian high society. The concept was then mothballed for one hundred years before reappearing in the 1970s as Dissociative Identity Disorder.) In both cases, psychiatrists have never been able to agree on what the disorder is, what its symptoms are, or whether it even exists. In both cases, heated debates over whether treatment does more harm than good, and even whether the "disorder" is actually a consequence of the "treatment," remain unresolved. And both disorders saw recent explosions in numbers of cases.

The idea that humans have something called an "identity" that can be pathologically "disordered" and put back into order with pharmaceutical products sold at a profit is now moving out beyond the confines of diagnoses that actually include the word *identity*. Peter Kramer began his ground-breaking *Listening to Prozac* with a discussion of a patient who insisted that without Prozac, "I am not myself."[13] More recently, in *Coming of Age on Zoloft*, Katherine Sharpe writes of being part of the first generation to begin long-term use of antidepressants while still teenagers:

> Worries about how antidepressants might affect the self are greatly magnified for people who begin using them in adolescence, before they've developed a stable, adult sense of self. Lacking a reliable conception of what it is to feel "like themselves," young people have no way to gauge the effects of the drugs on their developing personalities. Searching for identity—asking "Who am I?" and combing the inner and outer worlds for an answer that seems to fit—is the main developmental task of the teenage years. And for some young adults, the idea of taking a medication that could frustrate that search can become a discouraging, painful preoccupation.[14]

Note that depression is another disease that has ignited enormous controversy, features an expanding arsenal of new pharmaceutical products sold at enormous profit yet whose effects in the body are poorly understood, and has vague and confusing diagnostic criteria that continue to elude clarification. And here again profound debates continue among doctors who wonder if they are treating a "real" disease or making patients "better than well."[15]

John Hoberman, whose *Testosterone Dreams* is the only book-length scholarly work on hormone use in sports, has written thoughtfully of the role played by elite athletes as a sort of battering ram breaking down the social barriers to a new kind of medicine in which "the alteration of human physiology for non-therapeutic purposes is permissible" and "personal satisfaction legitimates medical treatment."[16] Note the similarity between the argument that "personal satisfaction legitimates medical treatment" and Harry Benjamin's argument that the request for sex-change surgery be used as the diagnostic criterion for the disease the surgery would cure.

Hoberman views elite athletes as "expendable role models" subjected to ritual tests in which they are expected to both break all previous records of human performance and "provide symbolic confirmation of the unchanging essence of human nature at a time when that very idea has been radically destabilized." The never-ending seesaw balancing their never-before-accomplished triumphs on one end and doping scandals on the other, pushes and pulls the culture into the new medical order: "Athlete-doctor relationships have anticipated the increasing client demand for restorative or enhancing medical services among ordinary people, who often expect hormone therapy to improve or extend their lives," and thus "the demand for hormone therapies has now achieved a momentum that is both unprecedented and unstoppable."[17]

Hoberman has a name for this new medical paradigm of practices, technologies, and rights: *client-centered libertarian medicine.* He calls it libertarian because "regulation becomes impossible once physicians allow patients—as some sports physicians have long allowed their athlete-clients—to specify their own pharmacological requirements so as to realize 'the patient's vision of human flourishing.'" The consequences, he argues, are profound: "The philosophical issues raised by enhancement procedures originate in the most basic questions about what it means to be a human being [and] challenge our sense of human identity. . . . The 'doping' of athletes with androgens and other hormones can thus be understood as one of the human enhancements that will precipitate an unprecedented crisis of human identity during the twenty-first century."[18]

Hacking described a loop between new scientific classifications of kinds of people and the way people who fall within the new classification become aware of being classified, experience that classification as a "way to be a person," and as a result "enhance and adjust what is true of them," triggering a change in the original classification and another trip around the loop. I wish to argue that in transgender medicine, a new dimension is added to this looping effect, for identity now feeds back into the loop of *classification and description* outlined by Hacking but also into a loop of *scientifically authorized technologies that affect the immediately visible physiology of our bodies to such an extent that we understand them to cause a change in our identity or sense of self.* The overlapping of the two loops create complex, interlocking dynamics that play out differently in the very different social spheres of the transgender community and professional sports.

Money plays a central role in both, but is cast quite differently. Professional athletes have plenty of money, enough money not only to buy hormones but to secure the services of doctors even if those services are viewed negatively by most medical authorities, banned by sports leagues, or even illegal. So getting health insurance to pay for the hormones is not an issue, and the question of whether they are sick is absent. In its place is the question of whether they are human, whether the records they set "count" as human. The athletes themselves are figuratively and—considering the effects of the drugs—literally torn apart by the intense conflicting pressures to break all previous records of human performance and "provide symbolic confirmation of the unchanging essence of human nature at a time when that very idea has been radically destabilized."

The money at stake in how the two loops play out in the transgender community is the money to pay for hormones. And the question that tears the community apart is not whether transgender people are human but whether they are sick. Are the hormones *medicine for treating an illness,* which should be covered by health insurance? Or, as Susan Stryker argues, are they a *technology you electively engage with* in order to realize a more complete version of yourself (in which case you can still demand health insurance coverage but the going will be far more difficult)? The claims are not just different but contradictory. Each undercuts the other, which accounts at least in part for the much-discussed anger and bitterness that have come to infuse these debates within the transgender community.

The tension between the *scientific classification and identity* loop and the *technology and identity* loop can be clearly seen in the tensions within the community over who is transgender. Does living with Gender Identity Disorder or Gender Dysphoria make you transgender whether or not you take hormones? That is the *scientific classification and identity* loop. Or do hormones constitute a necessary "rite of passage" to becoming transgender? That is the *technology and identity* loop.

Remember that the discourse of the trans community is not merely a *symptom* of these loops but a *component* in them. This is how those who fall within this new scientific classification are "enhancing and adjusting what is true of them." But the discourse is functioning simultaneously in both loops, one that loops back to medical diagnosis and one that loops back to medical technology.

The contradictory pressures of the two loops are precipitating Hoberman's "unprecedented crisis of human identity." Hacking, writing in 1999, suggested that if the two loops were to fuse into one the result would be "a world that no one can foresee."[19]

Transpeople are bringing that world into view. Professional athletes, the millions more using E or T, and the hundreds of millions more who are taking one of the growing number of pharmaceutical products for diagnoses that veer into classifications of kinds of people, are close behind. But transpeople make the link between classification, technology, and identity explicit.

From where I sit, I can see no turning back from this new world, but that doesn't mean its particulars are already determined. Where do we go from here? Will this new world be more or less democratic? Will power be highly concentrated or more equitably disbursed? Will the boundaries between the majority and those whose sexual or gendered behavior mark them as *other* be enforced harshly or gently?

I worry that so much of the queer community has placed its social and political bets on the claim that minuscule variations in the chemicals we are exposed to in the womb determine the details of our adult behavior down to career aptitudes, our choice of sexual partners, our sense of gender, the kinds of sexual foreplay we enjoy, and aspects of our dreams while asleep. If we really believe that brains are so "masculinized" and "feminized," then why *shouldn't* we prepare men and women for different career paths? And what about medical intervention at the fetal stage? If we really believe minute differences in prenatal chemical exposure determine who does what when we become adults, should we manipulate those exposures *in utero* to build a better society? This is what Maria New claims to already be doing.

What of race? Can research measuring the exposure differences between races be far off? If we really believe that homosexuality and gender identity can only be understood by measuring prenatal hormone exposure, why shouldn't we seek to understand the minute differences in prenatal hormone exposures between races? If there is a gay brain and a trans brain and a male brain and a female brain, is there a black brain and a white brain? What's to prevent a new Louis Berman from restating the Columbia professor's claim from the 1930s that "since these endocrines control not only physique and physiognomy, anatomic and functional minutiae, but also mind and behaviour, we are justified in putting down the white man's predominance on the planet to a greater all-around concentration in his blood of the omnipotent hormones"?[20]

The French philosopher Michel Foucault warned, "There is not, on the one side, a discourse of power, and opposite it, another discourse that runs counter to it. Discourses are tactical elements of blocks operating in the field of force relations [that can] circulate without changing their form from one strategy to another, opposing strategy."[21] Over the course of my own adult life, I have watched as the gay liberation movement morphed from a countercultural movement in which a highly marginalized community of *others* sought their place alongside the other radical movements of the day, into a movement led by mainstream professionals that prioritized the right to marry and serve in the military. As the transgender movement takes its turn moving from the social margins to the mainstream, will its tight interface with the hierarchies of power of the medical industry make its conservative turn even harder?

The queer community has made enormous strides in the past few decades, sweeping aside prejudices and oppressions that have caused enormous suffering for the generations that preceded us. This is a dazzling achievement. It is all the more disturbing, therefore, that this same community is the first to put forward a political position asserting that there are certain meanings of technology it is unacceptable to question. I would far prefer that we lead the way into a knowing, eyes-open discussion of our very real suffering, our very fallible technologies, our imperfect understanding of complex natural systems including the human body, and our mutually constitutive relationships of money and power, privilege and access, pathology and well-being. Doing so will allow us to make choices that take into account the costs of those choices. It isn't only the queers who are perhaps too much in love with technology and all the many wonderful things that it can do; we have all made choices and entered into bargains without carefully reckoning the costs that they will bring, to us and to the generations that follow us, as global warming and dozens of other ongoing disasters amply demonstrate.

In the opening lines of my introduction, I wrote that my hope is that this book will be useful for anyone who has taken estrogen or testosterone, or considered doing so, for any reason. And that when I began this project, my interest was more narrowly focused on making something useful for young people wondering if they should begin hormone treatment in order to undergo what has become known as "transitioning" between genders. And their families. And their friends. So, how might this social history of so-called sex hormones be useful?

First, I want to make explicit my position that, with one exception, there is nothing in this book from which one can conclude, "Yes, I should take so-called sex hormones," or "No, I should not." And this holds for everyone this book is written for, from queer youth to menopausal women to amateur and professional athletes to business executives to soldiers fighting foreign wars. And this holds for me as well. I am getting up toward sixty years of age. As I continue to age and my energy and libido diminish, will I look around at a world of men my age jumping over tennis nets and continuing to engage in sexual pursuits of their younger years and think *Why not?* There is nothing in this book to cause me to rule that out. And as I noted in the introduction, I already take antidepressants, drugs that also lead directly to the vexing morass of issues we have before us here. They are sold at a huge profit by corporations whose advertising has centered less on what the drugs actually do and more on selling the very idea that depression is a "real" disease, in much the same way that the makers of testosterone and estrogen products have focused more on selling the idea that these are the chemical essences of gender than on what the substances actually do.[22] I know all this but I still take them, because I experience my life as nearly unbearable without them.

My point is not whether to take the drugs or not, but to be aware that the bargain we enter into when we do is a very large and complex one, and knowing this history will help understanding all the implications of the bargain.

Anyone who is considering taking estrogen or testosterone should know that the major clinical studies of both long-term estrogen use (which was huge, one of the biggest clinical trials in history) and long-term testosterone use (which was tiny) were suspended when the side effects of the drugs were deemed so harmful that continuing the trial to conclusion was judged unethical.

Anyone who is considering taking estrogen or testosterone to either transition their gender (transgender), amplify their gender (men who wish to be more masculine or women who wish to be more feminine), or reclaim their gender (aging people) should know that the idea that testosterone is the chemical essence of maleness and estrogen the chemical essence of femaleness comes from research done in the earliest days of endocrinology, which was thoroughly debunked nearly a hundred years ago but has lived on primarily through massive advertising campaigns run by the most powerful pharmaceutical corporations.

Even our understanding of what constitutes the "side effects" as opposed to desired effects of these products is profoundly colored by this. For example, when men take testosterone their muscle mass increases, their testicles shrivel, and their breasts grow. If one begins from the assumption that testosterone is the chemical essence of masculinity, then the increase in muscle mass is the expected effect and the shriveled testicles and enlarged breasts are surprising "side effects" that require explanation. But if we drop that assumption and just view testosterone as one of a number of hormones that cause diverse and visible changes in the body, which are even today very poorly understood, there is no need to explain "surprising side effects." From the ancient Mediterranean down to the Enlightenment, testicles were considered the surest sign of masculinity. Growing boys were fed animal testicles to ensure their future masculinity. Maladies considered to affect only men were treated with testicle extract. But testosterone does not cause testicles to grow, and since today we believe testosterone to be the source of masculinity, big testicles are off the list of markers of masculinity.

Anyone who feels entirely confident of the set of beliefs and medical

practices that have recently become the medical standard for transgender care should at least be aware that these same chemical substances
have been at the center of previous beliefs and medical practices that had
spectacular ascents fueled at least in part by the demands of potential
patients who fervently believed that these new practices were medical
necessities which they required in the most urgent way. These beliefs and
practices then crashed and burned in an equally spectacular way, often
with the same population that formerly viewed them as a medical necessity later viewing them as harm inflicted on them at great cost.

Anyone who advocates for health insurance coverage for gender
"transitioning" should at least be aware of the acute tension and bitter
disagreement over whether or not transgender people are "sick." Think it
through. Which side are you taking? Are you arguing that transgender
people are sick in the same way that the guy who works in the Amazon
warehouse and is fighting his insurance company for coverage for a kidney transplant is sick? If yes, then do you consider homosexuals also to
be sick? If not, can you articulate why the L, G, and B are not sick yet
the T are?

Conversely, if you do not wish to argue that transgender people are
sick but you still want to advocate for health insurance coverage of transgender care, can you articulate why? Have you thought through the implications of the idea that there are people who are somehow "less than
sick" yet should still have the medical procedures they want covered
by health insurance? This new kind of "less than sick" yet insured person is at the center of what Hoberman calls client-centered libertarian
medicine, aimed at realizing "the patient's vision of human flourishing."
Hoberman thinks this will precipitate an unprecedented crisis of human identity. What do you think about that? Have you considered the
broader implications of the transition of "identity politics" from identities based on shared birth circumstances and shared life experience to
chemically constructed identities of one?

Note that every major advocacy organization in the LGBT community, from the most fringe to the most mainstream, from street protestors
to congressional lobbyists, and from organizations that see their con-
stituency as mostly or exclusively transgender to those that see their con-
stituency as mostly or exclusively lesbian, gay, or bisexual—all demand
health insurance for gender "transitioning." At this point it would be

essentially impossible for any organizations or individuals in the LGBT community to clearly say that they were not in favor of health insurance for gender "transitioning."

Anyone who would argue against health insurance for transgender care should know that the list of available technologies is expensive. If health insurance does not make these technologies available to those without the means to pay for them, there will be an increasingly visible divide in the transgender world between those whose appearances reveal that they were able to pay for more and those who could afford less. This will happen in any event, as it is extremely unlikely that insurance will ever cover all the available options, which continue to expand. So this visible class divide will become more pronounced one way or the other. But without health insurance it will become much more so.

I am painfully aware that there are many in my own community who will take offense when I put "transitioning" in scare quotes, as I have done throughout this book. This is not my intention and I mean no disrespect. But to take the scare quotes away would be to accept the claim that testosterone and estrogen are substances that cause gender to transition. And not only to accept the claim but to reinforce it through yet more repeated discourse. I believe we would all benefit from a greater awareness of how the political taboos we are so adamantly placing on language are at the point of censuring honest discussion of history and science.

A few paragraphs back I wrote that I was not making an argument for or against anyone taking hormones, with one exception. Before we end, I must deal that that one exception: giving hormone blockers to young children. This is not a case of someone having the right to decide whether or not to take hormones. Rather, this is a case of doctors and parents deciding on the child's behalf. Children as young as nine years old. Those who engage in this practice insist that they are not deciding anything for the child because they do not give them estrogen or testosterone to initiate a gender "transition." They claim that by instead giving the child hormone blockers, which will shut down the processes of puberty in the child's body, they are only giving the child time to reach an age when he or she can decide whether to "transition" or not. They further claim to be able to confidently diagnose "gender dysphoria" in children of such a young age, and distinguish it from homosexuality, which would be illegal to treat in the four states that have banned gay conversion therapy for minors.[23] Finally, they claim that confidence in the safety of this practice can be gained from casual medical observation of the children being treated.

There is nothing in this book that supports any of those claims. As I have noted several times, the adult transgender community itself is fiercely divided over who is and isn't transgender. If the adults can't work it out among themselves, on what basis can a doctor claim the ability to diagnose a child? Much more importantly, there is nothing in the history of endocrinology to suggest that we have enough knowledge of the endocrine system to predict with even a remote sort of accuracy the long-term consequences of such a dramatic intervention in the development of such a young person. To the contrary, everything suggests we do not. I have already mentioned that recent research has established that pubertal hormone production—the very processes being shut down in these children—plays a significant role in brain development, a role we see some consequences of but that we hardly understand. To believe otherwise is exactly the sort of unjustified medical and scientific chutzpah that has repeatedly led doctors into catastrophic "sex hormone" debacles.

Neither does this history support the idea that "sex hormones" and "hormone blockers" are such different technologies that are so well understood that one can ethically be administered to a child and one cannot. And the idea that administering "sex hormones" would constitute initiation of treatment, while delaying puberty for years would constitute only a delaying or postponing of treatment, is absurd. It fully buys into the idea that there is a thing called "gender transitioning" that is initiated by one set of hormone technologies, and that this is unique and special and utterly distinct from intervening in the endocrinological system in other ways.

Yes, gender has become medicalized in our culture to such an extent that an anguished nine-year-old who is deeply distressed about his own body can tearfully declare to his father that he needs "medical help." The pain for both the child and the parent in such a situation must be profound. If I were the parent in such a situation I would feel my heart being torn out. But there is no resolution to be found in treating such a child with drugs whose consequences are poorly understood, distributed across the entire body, and implicated in many crucial systems.

Amid all the vexing questions that the story told in this book raises, this is the only one that I find the story actually answers. We adults may experiment with these technologies as we wish. Deciding on their behalf to administer these technologies to children is wrong. I strongly suspect that in the near future it will be the next item to be added to the long list of "sex hormone" medical catastrophes.

Afterword

This is a short book written in conversational English. But it contains many ideas I have tried to express quite precisely, because they address matters for which small changes in meaning make a world of difference.

To make whatever discussion this book leads to as fruitful as possible, I would like to restate some of these very specific ideas.

People have the right to define themselves any way they want to. I do not define who anyone is—men or women, males or females, transgender, Ls or Gs or Bs or Ts—not in my life, not in my relationships, and not in this book.

Everyone who writes about any substantive social issue must somehow deal with the fact that many of the terms we commonly use to identify ourselves have multiple and often contradictory meanings. Many writers simply ignore that fact and write as if this was not a problem—as if everybody already agrees on the meanings of the words that they use. I wanted to write a book that uses ideas and words in rigorous and consistent ways. So I chose specific meanings and used them throughout, and identified them for the reader at the outset. But as I was careful to add, I make no claim that these are the only definitions, or the correct definitions.

In order to write this book, I present anecdotes which make no claim to be representative of a rigorous statistical sampling of opinion in the trans community. What I infer from these anecdotes is quite limited, and readers are free to draw their own conclusions. I don't claim all trans people speak or write that way; I don't even claim that most do.

My only claim is that enough people do so that it piqued my curiosity: if pharmaceutical hormone technology is so important, what is it? Is the history of this technology readily available to the queer community? I discovered it was not, and decided that writing such a book would be a good service to the queer community.

Beyond that, I would argue that anecdotal data is the only kind of data we have concerning these questions. The idea that we could use survey methodologies to determine in a rigorous way how trans people "really" think of themselves, or who trans people "really" are, assumes that we can define the right group of people to sample. In other words, it assumes we already have the definition we are looking for. That is a circular logic. Furthermore, as I note many times, these definitions are the subject of bitter dispute within the community of people who claim the transgender identity for themselves. Whose definition would we use to define the group of people we were going to survey? As I note in the book, the transgender historian Susan Stryker concludes that "there is no way of using the word [transgender] that doesn't offend some people by including them where they don't want to be included or excluding them from where they want to be included."

Moreover, these definitions change rapidly. So any survey would not only have to begin using one definition among many, but would only be one snapshot at one point in time of even that definition.

I have argued that "sex hormones" and our beliefs about them have become a central issue in the queer community. The fact that some people identify as transgender yet choose not to take hormones does not contradict this. In fact, the emergence of a group of people who claim this identity but choose not to take hormones is yet another example of how important hormones have become: it is noteworthy when people choose not to take them.

I also argue that, given how important this technology has become, we should educate ourselves about it.

However, I do *not* argue that hormones are what make transpeople trans. I explicitly avoid defining who transpeople "really are," or what makes transpeople trans. I *do* argue that the belief that hormones make transpeople trans is widely held. But I also argue that the idea that hormones are what make homosexuals homosexual and heterosexuals heterosexual is equally widespread, and even the idea that hormones are what make men men and women women. Transpeople are no different than anyone else in this regard.

My book is not a transgender history. The book is a social history of estrogen and testosterone. I do not tell the story of any person or group of persons. I tell the story of estrogen and testosterone. The questions I seek to answer are these: Were these substances discovered or invented? Where did the idea that they are the chemical essence of gender come from? For what other purposes have they been used? Who owns them? Who profits from their sale? What do they actually do in your body? What are the risks of long-term use?

One of the main points of this book is that beliefs about the hormones taken as pills or injections are closely connected to beliefs about the hormones we are all exposed to prenatally in the womb, and also the hormones we are exposed to in the food we eat and the environment in which we live. Given that these beliefs are so widely and deeply held, I suggest that it is worthwhile to review whether the science upon which these beliefs are based holds water. And I found that it does not. Not even close. That is one of the central threads in this book.

I also suggest that we should *at least notice* when beliefs that we hold to be important are used in ways we find abhorrent. The same bogus research we use today to claim that queers are "born that way" is what others use to claim that women's brains are less capable at math and science than male brains. One cannot claim that this "science" is rigorous when it is used for social goals we like and at the same time claim it is bunk when used for social goals we do not like.

The health effects of estrogen and testosterone remain poorly understood despite years of research involving millions of dollars and thousands of subjects. One thing that *is* clear is that there are consequences that take years to manifest, and are in any event difficult to discern. These substances affect growth (including the kinds of growth we call cancer), the brain, aging, and much more. Many studies suggest that the consequences of these substances vary depending on when in life they are taken, but again this is poorly understood. Many scientists now believe that environmental exposure to tiny amounts of synthetic chemicals that mimic the effects of hormones once they are inside our bodies can have terrible consequences, which certainly suggests caution when taking the substances in much larger doses deliberately.

This does not mean that no one should take them. Each person must balance the potential benefit with the potential harm. At a minimum, everyone considering taking them should know that the only long-term studies of the effects of these chemicals were shut down prior to completion when it was determined that the negative effects were so serious that it would have been unethical to continue the studies to completion. And these were studies of men and women who began to take hormones late in life, and were never even contemplating the extended duration of treatment many young transpeople face.

And we should be aware of inconsistencies in our thoughts in this regard. For example, it is difficult to reconcile the belief that children diagnosed as transgender should be given hormone blockers with the belief that Bisphenol A should be banned from plastic in children's toys.

This book is intended to begin a discussion, not end one. There is nothing here that is presented as the last or final word about anything. And anyway there is no last word to be had, especially now that technology is evolving at such a rapid pace. As it does, new spaces for the creation and adjudication of human identity will open.

This book is an invitation to think freely and critically about these new spaces: to learn their histories; to become informed about what is actually known and unknown about them medically; and to understand their economies. Technology does not fall from the sky. It is invented and developed and advertised and sold. People profit from those sales. These people are extremely powerful in our culture, and have an enormous interest in showcasing the benefits of their technology and hiding its dangers.

This book is not "anti-technology." There is no turning back to an imagined world before technology. But in order to maximize the happiness and minimize the suffering we will reap from all of this, we must walk into this new world with our eyes open, a quizzical expression, and a critical mind, examining each new option the way a cashier examines a hundred-dollar bill for signs of counterfeiting.

Notes

Introduction

1. Suzanne Goldenberg, "Why Women Are Poor at Science, by Harvard President," *Guardian* (London), January 18, 2005.

2. Tracy Stanton, "10 Big Brands Keep Pumping Out Big Bucks, with a Little Help from Price Hikes," *Fierce PharmaMarketing*, May 7, 2014, www.fiercepharmamarketing.com.

3. "Annual Testosterone Drug Revenue in the U.S. in 2013 and 2018," 2015, *Statista*, www.statista.com (based on a report by Global Industry Analysts, www.strategyr.com).

4. Author's interviews, October 2013 and February 2014.

5. For a superb and readable account of the worldwide spread of US psychiatric culture, see Ethan Watters, *Crazy Like Us: The Globalization of the American Psyche* (New York: Free Press, 2010).

6. Nelly Oudshoorn, *Beyond the Natural Body: An Archeology of Sex Hormones* (New York: Routledge, 1994); Anne Fausto-Sterling, *Sexing the Body: Gender Politics and the Construction of Sexuality* (New York: Basic Books, 2000); Barbara Seaman, *The Greatest Experiment Ever Performed on Women: Exploding the Estrogen Myth* (New York: Hyperion, 2003); Elizabeth Siegel Watkins, *The Estrogen Elixir: A History of Hormone Replacement Therapy in America* (Baltimore: Johns Hopkins University Press, 2007); John Hoberman, *Testosterone Dreams: Rejuvenation, Aphrodisia, Doping* (Berkeley: University of California Press, 2005); Chandak Sengoopta, *The Most Secret Quintessence of Life: Sex, Glands, and Hormones, 1850–1950* (Chicago: University of Chicago Press, 2006).

7. Zack Ford, "The Transgender Tipping Point," *Time*, June 9, 2014.

8. Leslie Feinberg, *Transgender Warriors: Making History from Joan of Arc to Dennis Rodman* (Boston: Beacon, 1996); Joanne Meyerowitz, *How Sex Changed: A History of Transsexuality in the United States* (Cambridge: Harvard University Press, 2002); Deborah Rudacille, *The Riddle of Gender: Science, Activism, and Transgender Rights* (New York: Pantheon, 2006); Susan Stryker, *Transgender History* (Berkeley: Seal Press, 2008); Susan Stryker and Steven Whittle, eds., *The Transgender Studies Reader* (New York: Routledge, 2006). Bernice L. Hausman's *Changing Sex: Transsexualism, Technology, and the Idea of Gender* (Durham, NC: Duke University Press, 1995) should also be mentioned here, although Hausman writes almost exclusively on sex reassignment surgery, not hormones.

9. Harry Benjamin, "The Late Professor Steinach," *New York Times*, June 3, 1944.

10. Christine Jorgensen, *Christine Jorgensen: A Personal Autobiography* (New York: Paul S. Eriksson, 1967), 71, 77; Paul de Kruif, *The Male Hormone* (New York: Harcourt, Brace, 1945).

11. Quoted in Sengoopta, *The Most Secret Quintessence of Life*, 100.

12. Oudshoorn, *Beyond the Natural Body*, 77.

13. "Monitor Gender Identity Watch as a Hate Group," an online petition started by the group Secular Women demanding that the Southern Poverty Law Center add the feminist group Gender Identity Watch to its list of hate groups operating in the United States, at www.change.org. Chase Strangio, "Call Her Caitlyn but Then Let's Move on to the Issues Affecting the Trans Community," June 1, 2015, www.aclu.org.

14. Hoberman, *Testosterone Dreams*, 4, 17.

15. Bob Ostertag, *Creative Life: Music, Politics, People, and Machines* (Champaign: Illinois University Press, 2009); Bob Ostertag, *People's Movements, People's Press: The Journalism of Social Justice Movements* (Boston: Beacon, 2006); Jane McAlevey with Bob Ostertag, *Raising Expectations (and Raising Hell): My Decade Fighting for the Labor Movement* (London: Verso, 2012); Anonymous, *The Yes Men: The True Story of the End of the World Trade Organization* (New York: Disinformation, 2004).

16. Quoted in Dave King and Richard Ekins, "Pioneers of Transgendering: The Life and Work of Virginia Prince," paper presented at the Gendys 2K Conference, University of Manchester, UK, September 2000, available at www.gender.org.uk; Virginia Prince, *The Transvestite and His Wife* (Los Angeles: Argyle, 1967).

17. Stryker, *Transgender History*, 24.

18. Justin Vivian Bond is both a longtime personal friend and a longtime collaborator of mine. V (the pronoun Justin Vivian prefers) sings on my *Fear No Love* CD, and, along with myself and Otomo Yoshihide, was in the group *PantyChrist*, which released one CD and toured Europe.

19. Justin Vivian Bond, "Mx Justin Vivian Bond: A User's Guide," http://justinbond.com.

20. As of this writing, the most recent high-profile transition from lesbian to transgender male is that of Chaz Bono, whose transition is the subject of a feature-length documentary, *Becoming Chaz* (2011).

21. Quoted in Rudacille, *The Riddle of Gender*, 59.

22. Christine Johnson, "Endocrine Disruptors and the Transgendered," March 27, 2002, Trans-Health.com; Scott P. Kerlin, "Prenatal Exposure to Diethylstilbestrol (DES) in Males and Gender-Related Disorders: Results from a 5-Year Study," paper presented at the International Behavioral Development Symposium, Minot, North Dakota, August 2005. For more recent research, see *TransAdvocate.org*, www.antijen.org/transadvocate.

23. Author's interview, August 29, 2011.

24. Author's interview, August 29, 2011; "Sam" is a pseudonym.

25. Philip A. Mackowiak, Steven S. Wasserman, and Myron M. Levine, "A Critical Appraisal of 98.6°F, the Upper Limit of the Normal Body Temperature, and Other Legacies of Carl Reinhold August Wunderlich," *Journal of the American Medical Association* 268.12 (1992): 1578–80.

26. Fausto-Sterling, *Sexing the Body*, 169.

1. Before Pharmaceuticals

1. Jean D. Wilson and Claus Roehrborn, "Long-Term Consequences of Castration in Men: Lessons from the Skoptzy and the Eunuchs of the Chinese and Ottoman Courts," *Journal of Clinical Endocrinology and Metabolism* 84.12 (1999): 4324–25.

2. David M. Friedman, *A Mind of Its Own: A Cultural History of the Penis* (New York: Penguin, 2001), 82.

3. Nelly Oudshoorn, *Beyond the Natural Body: An Archeology of Sex Hormones* (New York: Routledge, 1994), 17.

4. David Hamilton, *The Monkey Gland Affair* (London: Chatto and Windus, 1986), 15.

5. R. V. Short, "The Discovery of the Ovaries," in *The Ovary*, ed. Solomon Zuckerman and Barbara J. Weir, 2nd ed., vol. 1 (London: Academic Press, 1977), 1–39, quotation on 1.

6. Quoted in Chandak Sengoopta, *The Most Secret Quintessence of Life: Sex, Glands, and Hormones, 1850–1950* (Chicago: University of Chicago Press, 2006), 14.

7. Walter Bernardi, "The Controversy on Animal Electricity in Eighteenth-Century Italy: Galvani, Volta, and Others," in *Nuova Voltiana: Studies on Volta and His Times*, vol. 1, ed. Fabio Bevilacqua and Lucio Fregonese (Milan: Hoepli, 2000), 101–14.

8. Edward Hare, "The History of 'Nervous Disorders' from 1600 to 1840, and a Comparison with Modern Views," *British Journal of Psychiatry* 159.1 (1991): 37–45.

9. Erica R. Freeman, David A. Bloom, and Edward J. McGuire, "A Brief History of Testosterone," *Journal of Urology* 165.2 (2001): 371–73.

10. Friedman, *A Mind of Its Own*, 261.

11. John Henderson, "Ernest Starling and 'Hormones': An Historical Commentary," *Journal of Endocrinology* 184.1 (2005): 5–10.

12. Andrew Scull, *Hysteria: The Biography* (Oxford: Oxford University Press, 2009), 14. See also Helen King, "Once Upon a Text: Hysteria from Hippocrates," in *Hysteria beyond Freud,* ed. Sander L. Gilman et al. (Berkeley: University of California Press, 1993), 3–90.

13. Quoted in Rachel P. Maines, *The Technology of Orgasm: "Hysteria," the Vibrator, and Women's Sexual Satisfaction* (Baltimore: Johns Hopkins University Press, 1999), 27.

14. Ibid., 5, 38.

15. Quoted in Carroll Smith-Rosenberg, *Disorderly Conduct: Visions of Gender in Victorian America* (Oxford: Oxford University Press, 1985), 201.

16. D. A. B. Young, "Florence Nightingale's Fever," *British Medical Journal* 311.1 (1995): 1697–1700.

17. Scull, *Hysteria,* 29.

18. Ibid., 75; John Studd, "Ovariotomy for Menstrual Madness and Premenstrual Syndrome—19th Century History and Lessons for Current Practice," *Gynecological Endocrinology* 22.8 (2006): 411–15.

19. Scull, *Hysteria,* 88–89.

20. Studd, "Ovariotomy," 413; Scull, *Hysteria,* 90.

21. Studd, "Ovariotomy," 413.

22. Ibid., 412.

23. Elizabeth Siegel Watkins, *The Estrogen Elixir: A History of Hormone Replacement Therapy in America* (Baltimore: Johns Hopkins University Press, 2007), 17.

24. Scull, *Hysteria,* 92.

25. Freeman, Bloom, and McGuire, "History of Testosterone," 371.

26. Charles-Édouard Brown-Séquard, *The Elixir of Life: Dr. Brown-Séquard's Own Account of His Famous Alleged Remedy for Debility and Old Age . . .* , ed. Newell Dunbar (Boston: J. G. Cupples, 1889), 24–25, 30–32, 37.

27. Ibid., 43, 116.

28. Arnold Kahn, "Regaining Lost Youth: The Controversial and Colorful Beginnings of Hormone Replacement Therapy in Aging," *Journal of Gerontology* 60A.2 (2005): 145.

29. Watkins, *The Estrogen Elixir,* 14.

30. "Testicle and Ovary Endocrine Therapy," *Journal of the American Medical Association* 75.23 (1920): 1598; see also John Hoberman, *Testosterone Dreams: Rejuvenation, Aphrodisia, Doping* (Berkeley: University of California Press, 2005), 34.

31. Arthur F. W. Hughes, "A History of Endocrinology," *Journal of the History of Medicine and Allied Sciences* 32.3 (1977): 292–313.

32. Hamilton, *The Monkey Gland Affair*, 18.

33. Sengoopta, *The Most Secret Quintessence*, 38; Hoberman, *Testosterone Dreams*, 37.

34. Antony O. W. Stretton, "The First Sequence: Fred Sanger and Insulin," *Genetics* 162.2 (2002): 527–32.

35. Sengoopta, *The Most Secret Quintessence*, 42, 58.

36. Ibid., 60–65.

37. Quoted in Anne Fausto-Sterling, *Sexing the Body: Gender Politics and the Construction of Sexuality* (New York: Basic Books, 2000), 161.

38. Quoted ibid., 165.

39. See Rebecca M. Jordan-Young, *Brain Storm: The Flaws in the Science of Sex Differences* (Cambridge: Harvard University Press, 2011). See also Fausto-Sterling, *Sexing the Body*.

40. Rainer Herrn, "On the History of Biological Theories of Homosexuality," *Journal of Homosexuality* 28.1–2 (1995): 45.

41. Quoted ibid.

42. Hubert Kennedy, *Karl Heinrich Ulrichs: Pioneer of the Modern Gay Movement* (San Francisco: Peremptory Publications, 2002), 7. Ulrichs is generally thought to be the first self-proclaimed Urning (his terminology; the word "homosexual" did not come until later) to publicly advocate for the rights of Urnings.

43. Herrn, "On the History of Biological Theories of Homosexuality," 34.

44. Chandak Sengoopta, "Glandular Politics: Experimental Biology, Clinical Medicine, and Homosexual Emancipation in Fin-de-Siècle Central Europe," *Isis* 89.3 (1998): 445–73, quotation on 452.

45. Magnus Hirschfeld, *The Homosexuality of Men and Women* (1914), trans. Michael A. Lombardi-Nash (Amherst, NY: Prometheus, 2000). For Hirschfeld's discussion of the monthly menstruation of homosexual men, see 170–71.

46. Mel Gordon, *Voluptuous Panic: The Erotic World of Weimar Berlin,* 2nd ed. (Port Townsend, WA: Feral House, 2006), 84–86.

47. Herrn, "On the History of Biological Theories of Homosexuality," 38.

48. Sengoopta, "Glandular Politics," 465.

49. Ibid., 468.

50. Sengoopta, *The Most Secret Quintessence*, 79–80.

51. Herrn, "On the History of Biological Theories of Homosexuality," 46, 48; Sengoopta, *The Most Secret Quintessence,* 81.

52. Sengoopta, *The Most Secret Quintessence*, 83.

53. Quoted in Christopher Turner, "Vasectomania, and Other Cures for Sloth," *Cabinet* no. 29 (2008), www.cabinetmagazine.org.

54. "Gland Treatment Spreads in America," *New York Times*, April 8, 1923.

55. Quoted in Sengoopta, *The Most Secret Quintessence*, 84.

56. Turner, "Vasectomania."

57. Gertrude Atherton, *Black Oxen* (New York: A. L. Burt, 1923).

58. Turner, "Vasectomania."

59. Hamilton, *The Monkey Gland Affair*, 66.

60. Quoted in Watkins, *The Estrogen Elixir*, 30.

61. Hamilton, *The Monkey Gland Affair*, 62, 91–92; Max Thorek, *The Human Testis: Its Gross Anatomy, Histology, Physiology, Pathology, with Particular Reference to Its Endocrinology* (Philadelphia: J. B. Lippincott, 1924).

62. Hamilton, *The Monkey Gland Affair*, 34–35.

63. Chandak Sengoopta, "Tales from the Vienna Labs: The Eugen Steinach–Harry Benjamin Correspondence," *Favourite Edition: Newsletter of the Friends of the Rare Book Room* (New York Academy of Medicine Library) 2 (Spring 2000): 5.

64. Ethan Blue, "The Strange Career of Leo Stanley: Remaking Manhood and Medicine at San Quentin State Penitentiary, 1913–1951," *Pacific Historical Review* 78.2 (2009): 228, 211; Hamilton, *The Monkey Gland Affair*, 68.

65. Sengoopta, "Glandular Politics," 98; Hamilton, *The Monkey Gland Affair*, 68.

66. Quoted in Blue, "The Strange Career of Leo Stanley," 231.

67. Quoted in Christer Nordlund, "Endocrinology and Expectations in 1930s America: Louis Berman's Ideas on New Creations in Human Beings," *British Journal for the History of Science* 40.1 (2007): 93.

68. Quoted in Sengoopta, *The Most Secret Quintessence*, 73.

69. Hamilton, *The Monkey Gland Affair*, 112–18.

70. Ibid., 125.

71. Ibid., 104.

72. "Dr. Eugen Steinach," *New York Times*, May 16, 1944.

73. Harry Benjamin, "The Late Professor Steinach," *New York Times*, June 3, 1944.

2. The "Male Sex Hormone" and the Testosterone Gold Rush

1. Chandak Sengoopta, *The Most Secret Quintessence of Life: Sex, Glands, and Hormones, 1850–1950* (Chicago: University of Chicago Press, 2006), 162; Nelly Oudshoorn, *Beyond the Natural Body: An Archeology of Sex Hormones* (New York: Routledge, 1994), 53.

2. Ibid., 64–76.

3. Sengoopta, *The Most Secret Quintessence*, 137.

4. Oudshoorn, *Beyond the Natural Body*, 24–29.

5. Sengoopta, *The Most Secret Quintessence*, 143–44.

6. Quoted in Oudshoorn, *Beyond the Natural Body*, 17.

7. Paul de Kruif, *The Male Hormone* (New York: Harcourt, Brace, 1945), 188.

8. Oudshoorn, *Beyond the Natural Body*, 78.

9. Quoted ibid., 78, emphasis added.

10. Ibid., 78.

11. Christoph Gunkel, "Medicating a Madman: A Sober Look at Hitler's Health," *Der Spiegel International*, February 4, 2010; *Business Week* quoted in John Hoberman, *Testosterone Dreams: Rejuvenation, Aphrodisia, Doping* (Berkeley: University of California Press, 2005), 2–3; "Testosterone," *Time*, September 23, 1935.

12. Quoted in Sengoopta, *The Most Secret Quintessence*, 187.

13. Quoted ibid., 189.

14. Ibid., 188.

15. Hoberman, *Testosterone Dreams*, 110–11.

16. De Kruif, *The Male Hormone*, 127.

17. Hoberman, *Testosterone Dreams*, 98–99; Sengoopta, *The Most Secret Quintessence*, 189.

18. Andrew Hodges, *Alan Turing: The Enigma* (New York: Walker, 2000).

19. Bob Ostertag, *People's Movements, People's Press: The Journalism of Social Justice Movements* (Boston: Beacon, 2006), 73–75.

20. Hoberman, *Testosterone Dreams*, 106–8.

21. Albin Krebs, "Dr. Paul de Kruif, Popularizer of Medical Exploits, Is Dead," *New York Times*, March 2, 1971.

22. "Virility Prolonged," *Time*, May 28, 1945.

23. De Kruif, *The Male Hormone*, 139, 25, 23, 19, 86–87, 107, and pretty much any page in the book.

24. Hoberman, *Testosterone Dreams*, 142–43.

25. Quoted ibid., 75 (emphasis added), from H. S. Rubenstein, H. D. Shapiro, and Walter Freeman, "The Treatment of Morbid Sex Craving with the Aid of Testosterone Propionate," *American Journal of Psychiatry* 97.3 (November 1940): 703–10.

26. This analysis of the failure of testosterone marketing in the mid-twentieth century draws on Hoberman, *Testosterone Dreams*.

3. The "Female Sex Hormone," the Goddess of Fortune

1. Nelly Oudshoorn, *Beyond the Natural Body: An Archeology of Sex Hormones* (New York: Routledge, 1994), 87, 43.

2. Elizabeth Siegel Watkins, *The Estrogen Elixir: A History of Hormone Replacement Therapy in America* (Baltimore: Johns Hopkins University Press, 2007), 61.

3. Oudshoorn, *Beyond the Natural Body*, 88–91.

4. Barbara Seaman, *The Greatest Experiment Ever Performed on Women: Exploding the Estrogen Myth* (New York: Hyperion, 2003), 43.

5. Ibid., 13.

6. Ibid., 35.

7. Nancy Langston, *Toxic Bodies: Hormone Disruptors and the Legacy of DES* (New Haven: Yale University Press, 2010), 31–33.

8. Seaman, *The Greatest Experiment*, 38, 14.

9. Helen Haberman, "Help for Women over Forty," *Reader's Digest*, November 1941.

10. Langston, *Toxic Bodies*, 28–29.

11. Seaman, *The Greatest Experiment*, 9, 55–56, 49.

12. All of the quotations and details concerning William Masters in this section are from Watkins, *The Estrogen Elixir*, 36–41.

13. Thomas Maier, "Can Psychiatrists Really 'Cure' Homosexuality?," *Scientific American*, April 22, 2009.

14. Robert Wilson, *Feminine Forever* (New York: M. Evans, 1968).

15. Quoted in Seaman, *The Greatest Experiment*, 58.

16. Quoted ibid., 51.

17. Langston, *Toxic Bodies*, 48–53.

18. Watkins, *The Estrogen Elixir*, 26; Seaman, *The Greatest Experiment*, 37, 73.

19. Joyce M. Lee and Joel D. Howell, "Tall Girls: The Social Shaping of a Medical Therapy," *Archives of Pediatric and Adolescent Medicine* 160.10 (2006): 1035–39.

20. Langston, *Toxic Bodies*, 75.

21. Ibid., 69.

22. Elizabeth Siegel Watkins, *On the Pill: A Social History of Oral Contraceptives, 1950–1970* (Baltimore: Johns Hopkins University Press, 1998).

23. Ibid., 22.

24. Quoted in Seaman, *The Greatest Experiment,* 58.

25. For a nuanced analysis see Watkins, *On the Pill.*

26. Watkins, *The Estrogen Elixir,* 54, 83.

4. The Estrogen Mess

1. Elizabeth Siegel Watkins, *The Estrogen Elixir: A History of Hormone Replacement Therapy in America* (Baltimore: Johns Hopkins University Press, 2007), 187.

2. Elizabeth Siegel Watkins, *On the Pill: A Social History of Oral Contraceptives, 1950–1970* (Baltimore: Johns Hopkins University Press, 1998), 118.

3. Ibid., 5.

4. Nancy Langston, *Toxic Bodies: Hormone Disruptors and the Legacy of DES* (New Haven: Yale University Press, 2010), 98–100.

5. Watkins, *The Estrogen Elixir,* 130.

6. Fuller Albright, Esther Bloomberg, and Patricia H. Smith, "Postmenopausal Osteoporosis," *Transactions of the Association of American Physicians* 55 (1940): 298–305.

7. Watkins, *The Estrogen Elixir,* 176, 154, 166.

8. Quoted ibid., 171.

9. Jane Fonda, *Women Coming of Age* (New York: Simon and Schuster, 1986).

10. Watkins, *The Estrogen Elixir,* 245, 254 (quotation).

11. Gail Sheehy, *The Silent Passage: Menopause* (New York: Pocket Books, 1993), 63.

12. Watkins, *The Estrogen Elixir,* 130.

13. Ibid., 246–47, 253.

14. Ibid., 148, 246.

15. Jane Allin, "Pfizer Consigns PMU Horses to Killing Fields of Asia," *Tuesday's Horse,* March 31, 2012, tuesdayshorse.wordpress.com.

16. "Horse Urine a Profitable Industry," BON TV China, May 22, 2012, www.bon.tv/Biz-Wire.

17. Quoted in Watkins, *The Estrogen Elixir,* 178.

18. Ibid., 215.

19. JoAnn E. Manson et al., "Menopausal Hormone Therapy and Health Outcomes during the Intervention and Extended Poststopping Phases of the Women's Health Initiative Randomized Trials," *Journal of the American Medical Association* 310.13 (2013): 1353–68, available at http://jama.jamanetwork.com.

20. Sindell v. Abbott Laboratories (1980) 26 Cal. 3d 588.

21. Robert N. Hoover et al., "Adverse Health Outcomes in Women Exposed in Utero to Diethylstilbestrol," *New England Journal of Medicine* 365.1 (2011): 1304–14.

22. Scott P. Kerlin, "Prenatal Exposure to Diethylstilbestrol (DES) in Males and Gender-Related Disorders: Results from a 5-Year Study," paper presented at the International Behavioral Development Symposium, Minot, North Dakota, August 2005.

23. US Food and Drug Administration, "Update on Bisphenol A (BPA) for Use in Food Contact Applications," January 2010, www.fda.gov.

5. The Testosterone Comeback

1. Luke Harding, "Forgotten Victims of East German Doping Take Their Battle to Court," *Guardian* (London), October 31, 2005.

2. Alan Nothnagle, "East German Doping Scandal Refuses to Die," *Salon,* August 19, 2009, www.salon.com.

3. Sigfrid Schwarz, Dieter Onken, and Alfred Schubert, "The Steroid Story of Jenapharm: From the Late 1940s to the Early 1970s," *Steroids* 64.7 (1999): 439–45.

4. Jere Longman, "East German Steroids' Toll: 'They Killed Heidi,'" *New York Times,* January 26, 2004.

5. Shaun Assael, *Steroid Nation: Juiced Home Run Totals, Anti-Aging Miracles, and a Hercules in Every High School—The Secret History of America's True Drug Addiction* (New York: ESPN Books, 2007), 7–8.

6. Ibid., 16–19, 48–49.

7. Lloyd D. Johnston et al., "Monitoring the Future: National Results on Adolescent Drug Use" (Ann Arbor: Institute for Social Research, University of Michigan, 2011), www.monitoringthefuture.org.

8. "Join the Anti-Aging Movement," www.a4m.com.

9. Shannon Pettypiece, "Testosterone Chases Viagra in Libido Race as Doctors Fret," *Bloomberg.com,* May 1, 2012.

10. John Hoberman, *Testosterone Dreams: Rejuvenation, Aphrodisia, Doping* (Berkeley: University of California Press, 2005), 123.

11. Sabrina Tavernise and Andrew Pollack, "Aid to Women, or Bottom Line? Advocates Split on Libido Pill," *New York Times,* June 13, 2015; Anne Skomorowsky, "Five Studies: Does Flibanserin Provide Real Sexual Benefits for Women?" *Pacific Standard,* September 30, 2015.

12. Nicholas Bakalar, "Prescription Drug Use Soared in Past Decade," *New York Times,* October 18, 2010.

13. Andrew Sullivan, "The He Hormone," *New York Times,* April 2, 2000.

14. Matthew Arnold, "DTC Report: Flat Is the New Up," *Medical Marketing and Media,* March 15, 2010, www.mmm-online.com.

15. On the amount spent by Abbott and the creation of the website, see "Demand Booms for 'Low T' Therapy," *Indianapolis Star,* May 6, 2012.

16. www.mens-sexual-health.org/newsletter/may03.html.

17. Pettypiece, "Testosterone Chases Viagra."

18. Author's Google searches done in May 2012.

19. Pettypiece, "Testosterone Chases Viagra."

20. Quoted in Elizabeth Siegel Watkins, *On the Pill: A Social History of Oral Contraceptives, 1950–1970* (Baltimore: Johns Hopkins University Press, 2001), 45.

21. Frederick C. W. Wu et al., "Identification of Late-Onset Hypogonadism in Middle-Aged and Elderly Men," *New England Journal of Medicine* 363.1 (2010): 123–35; W. J. Bremner, "Testosterone Deficiency and Replacement in Older Men" (editorial), ibid., 189–91; Shehzad Basaria et al., "Adverse Events Associated with Testosterone Administration," ibid., 109–22.

22. "The Lowdown on 'Low T,'" *UC Berkeley Wellness Letter,* May 2011, www.berkeleywellness.com.

23. Susan Donaldson James, "Police Juice Up on Steroids to Get 'Edge' on Criminals," *ABC News,* October 18, 2007, http://abcnews.go.com.

24. Bernard Mallee, "Who's on Testosterone?," *New Statesman,* July 7, 2003.

25. Hoberman, *Testosterone Dreams,* 285; Arlene Weintraub, "Testosterone Is Sure Looking Virile," *Bloomberg Businessweek,* November 9, 2009; Shannon Pettypiece, "Are Testosterone Drugs the Next Viagra?," *Bloomberg Businessweek,* May 10, 2012.

26. John Carroll, "Endo Gets Green Light for New Testosterone Gel," *Fierce Biotech,* December 30, 2010, www.fiercebiotech.com.

27. Ed Silverman, "Low T or High Risk? Testosterone Treatments and Heart Attacks," *Forbes,* January 29, 2014; Elisabeth Rosenthal, "A Push to Sell Testosterone Gels Troubles Doctors," *New York Times,* October 15, 2013.

6. "Sex Hormones" Redux—Not Yours, Your Mother's

1. Rainer Herrn, "On the History of Biological Theories of Homosexuality," *Journal of Homosexuality* 28.1–2 (1995): 44.

2. C. H. Phoenix, R. W. Goy, A. A. Gerall, and W. C. Young, "Organizing Action of Pre-natally Administered Testosterone Propionate on the Tissues Mediating Mating Behavior in the Female Guinea Pig," *Endocrinology* 65.1 (1959): 369–82.

3. John Money, "Hermaphroditism: An Inquiry into the Nature of a Human Paradox" (PhD diss., Harvard University, 1952).

4. Simone de Beauvoir, *The Second Sex,* trans. H. M. Parshley (1952; New York: Vintage, 1989), 267.

5. John Money and Anke Ehrhardt, *Man and Woman, Boy and Girl* (Baltimore: Johns Hopkins University Press, 1972).

6. Quoted in Deborah Rudacille, *The Riddle of Gender: Science, Activism, and Transgender Rights* (New York: Pantheon, 2006), 134.

7. Diamond was not, however, among the signatories of the paper.

8. Milton Diamond and H. Keith Sigmundson, "Sex Reassignment at Birth: A Long Term Review and Clinical Implications," *Archives of Pediatric and Adolescent Medicine* 151 (March 1997): 298–304.

9. John Colapinto, *As Nature Made Him: The Story of a Boy Who Was Raised as a Girl* (New York: HarperCollins, 2001); Rebecca M. Jordan-Young, *Brain Storm: The Flaws in the Science of Sex Differences* (Cambridge: Harvard University Press, 2011), 75.

10. Joanne Meyerowitz, *How Sex Changed: A History of Transsexuality in the United States* (Cambridge: Harvard University Press, 2002), 132.

11. Ibid., 122.

12. Rudacille, *The Riddle of Gender,* 122.

13. Meyerowitz, *How Sex Changed,* 222.

14. Rudacille, *The Riddle of Gender,* 125.

15. Meyerowitz, *How Sex Changed,* 176.

16. Ibid., 119–20.

17. Arthur D. Schwabe, David H. Solomon, Robert J. Stoller, and John P. Burnham, "Pubertal Feminization in a Genetic Male with Testicular Atrophy and Normal Urinary Gonadotropin," *Journal of Clinical Endocrinology and Metabolism* 22.8 (1962): 839–45.

18. More specifically, Money was a psychologist while Stoller was a psychiatrist, but both were mental health professionals working among endocrinologists.

19. Ibid., 844.

20. Harold Garfinkel, *Studies in Ethnomethodology* (Englewood Cliffs, NJ: Prentice-Hall, 1967), 286.

21. Robbie Sutton and Karen Douglas, *Social Psychology* (New York: Palgrave Macmillan, 2013), 360.

22. Garfinkel, *Studies in Ethnomethodology.* For an excellent account of Agnes's encounter

with Garfinkel see Joanne Finkelstein, *The Art of Self Invention: Image and Identity in Popular Visual Culture* (London: I. B. Taurus, 2007), 50–60.

23. Garfinkel, *Studies in Ethnomethodology,* 119.

24. Schwabe et al., "Pubertal Feminization"; Meyerowitz, *How Sex Changed,* 160.

25. Quoted in Meyerowitz, *How Sex Changed,* 161.

26. *Sylvester: Mighty Real* (documentary promo), dir. Tim Smyth (2002).

27. Jon K. Meyer and John E. Hoopes, "The Gender Dysphoria Syndromes: A Position on So-Called 'Transsexualism,'" *Plastic and Reconstructive Surgery* 54.4 (1974): 444–51. Quoted in Meyerowitz, *How Sex Changed,* 266.

28. Meyerowitz, *How Sex Changed,* 267.

29. Quoted in Jane E. Brody, "Benefits of Transsexual Surgery Disputed," *New York Times,* October 2, 1979.

30. "Sex Change at Stanford: Historical and Personal Perspectives on Stanford's Pioneering Gender Dysphoria Program, 1968–Present," forum presentation, Stanford University, April 13, 2000.

7. Brain Organization Theory

1. Quoted in Rebecca M. Jordan-Young, *Brain Storm: The Flaws in the Science of Sex Differences* (Cambridge: Harvard University Press, 2011), 31.

2. Ibid., 32–33.

3. John Money and Anke Ehrhardt, *Man and Woman, Boy and Girl* (Baltimore: Johns Hopkins University Press, 1972).

4. Jordan-Young, *Brain Storm,* 33.

5. Ibid., 36.

6. Ibid., 4–5.

7. Ibid., 5.

8. The phrase "female soul in a male body" was first published in 1865 by the queer rights pioneer Karl-Heinrich Ulrichs, who felt it sufficiently important to warrant translation into Latin: *anima muliebris virili corpore inclusa.* Hubert Kennedy, "Karl Heinrich Ulrichs: First Theorist of Homosexuality," in *Science and Homosexualities,* ed. Vernon Rosario (New York: Routledge, 1997), 26–27.

9. Jordan-Young, *Brain Storm,* xii.

10. Quoted ibid., 27.

11. Susan Stryker, *Transgender History* (Berkeley: Seal Press, 2008), 24.

12. Jordan-Young, *Brain Storm,* 234–36.

13. Ibid., 116.

14. Ibid., 132.

15. Ibid., 109.

16. Quoted ibid., 151.

17. Ibid., 159–60.

18. For an excellent history of how homosexuality was understood in pre–World War II America, see George Chauncey, *Gay New York: Gender, Urban Culture, and the Making of the Gay Male World, 1890–1940* (New York: Basic Books, 1995).

19. Craig A. Williams, *Roman Homosexuality: Ideologies of Masculinity in Classical Antiquity* (Oxford: Oxford University Press, 1999), 3.

20. Jordan-Young, *Brain Storm,* 228.

21. Maria Paul, "Clinicians Attempt to Prenatally Prevent Homosexuality" (press release),

Northwestern University, July 1, 2010; Alice Dreger, Ellen K. Feder, and Anne Tamar-Mattis, "Preventing Homosexuality (and Uppity Women) in the Womb?," *Bioethics Forum* (Hastings Center), June 29, 2010, www.thehastingscenter.org/Bioethicsforum.

22. Shari Roan, "Medical Treatment Carries Possible Side Effect of Limiting Homosexuality," *Los Angeles Times,* August 15, 2010; Sharon Begley, "The Anti-Lesbian Drug," *Newsweek,* July 2, 2010; Jacob M. Appel, "Tempest in a Womb: What's Wrong with Preventing (or Promoting) Homosexuality in Utero?," *Huffington Post,* July 22, 2010.

23. "Prenatal Treatment of Classic CAH with Dexamethasone: Pro vs. Con," *Endocrine News,* April 2008.

24. Gilbert H. Herdt and Julian Davidson, "The Sambia 'Turnim-Man': Sociocultural and Clinical Aspects of Gender Formation in Male Pseudohermaphrodites with 5-Alpha-Reductase Deficiency in Papua New Guinea," *Archives of Sexual Behavior* 117.11 (1988): 33–56.

25. The controversy surrounding New also includes the question of whether her patients were informed that this use of dexamethasone was off-label, whether they were informed of possible side effects, and perhaps most importantly whether her practice constitutes the sort of human medical research that by law should be done under the oversight of an Institutional Review Board (IRB). These are serious concerns; indeed, since I do not find the argument that dexamethasone reduces homosexuality to be convincing, I consider these other concerns to be the *more* serious part of the controversy.

26. Saroj Nimkarn and Maria I. New, "Congenital Adrenal Hyperplasia Due to 21-Hydroxylase Deficiency," *Annals of the New York Academy of Sciences* 1192 (2010): 5–11.

27. Heino F. L. Meyer-Bahlburg, Curtis Dolezal, Susan W. Baker, and Maria I. New, "Sexual Orientation in Women with Classical or Non-Classical Congenital Adrenal Hyperplasia as a Function of Degree of Prenatal Androgen Excess," *Archives of Sexual Behavior* 37.1 (2008): 85–99. All quotations in the remainder of the section are from this article.

28. There is actually a scale for describing the range of genital ambiguity (called the Prader scale), but Meyer-Bahlburg and New do not provide information on where their research subjects fall on this scale.

29. Stephen Jay Gould, *The Mismeasure of Man* (1981), rev. and exp. ed. (New York: Norton, 1996), 53.

30. Ibid., 20.

31. Ibid., 56–57.

32. Ibid., 60, 57.

33. Ibid., 105–6.

34. Ibid., 72.

35. Ibid., 54.

36. Ibid., 106.

8. The Contemporary Landscape

1. Quoted in Rainer Hernn, "On the History of Biological Theories of Homosexuality," *Journal of Homosexuality* 28.1–2 (1995): 45.

2. Quoted in Joanne Meyerowitz, *How Sex Changed: A History of Transsexuality in the United States* (Cambridge: Harvard University Press, 2002), 161.

3. "Standards of Care for the Health of Transsexual, Transgender, and Gender-Nonconforming People," version 7 (World Professional Association of Transgender Health, 2012), quotations on 34. Available at www.wpath.org.

4. Margie Mason, "Thailand's Sex-Change Industry," *Seattle Times,* September 3, 2006.

5. Meyerowitz, *How Sex Changed,* 183.

6. All quotes from Iranian sources are from Tanaz Eshaghian's stunning 2008 documentary film, *Be Like Others.*

7. Multiple interviews by the author.

8. Author's interview, June 8, 2011.

9. Author's interview, March 22, 2012.

10. Ibid., 57, 96.

11. John Hoberman, *Testosterone Dreams: Rejuvenation, Aphrodisia, Doping* (Berkeley: University of California Press, 2005), 14.

12. Quoted ibid., 199–200.

13. Author's interview, June 7, 2011.

14. Beth Schwartzapfel, "How Norman Spack Transformed the Way We Treat Transgender Children," *Boston Phoenix,* August 8, 2012.

15. Cheryl L. Sisk and Julia L. Zehr, "Pubertal Hormones Organize the Adolescent Brain and Behavior," *Frontiers in Neuroendocrinology* 26.3–4 (2005): 163–74.

Conclusion

1. "'Empowering, So Brave': Trans Activists Praise Chelsea Manning, Raise Fears over Prison Conditions," *Democracy Now,* August 23, 2013.

2. Distribution of material considered obscene through the US postal system was legally forbidden. Since post–World War II queer activists relied on the mail to distribute their publications, this law effectively criminalized their work. Novelists and journalists writing for major newspapers had ways to distribute their writing other than the post office. Bob Ostertag, *People's Movements, People's Press: The Journalism of Social Justice Movements* (Boston: Beacon, 2006), 73–75.

3. Rodger Streitmatter, *Unspeakable: The Rise of the Gay and Lesbian Press in America* (Boston: Faber and Faber, 1995).

4. In the words of the Combahee River Collective, whose "Statement" is generally credited as the first published articulation of identity politics, "the synthesis of these oppressions creates the conditions of our lives." "The Combahee River Collective Statement," in *Home Girls: A Black Feminist Anthology,* ed. Barbara Smith (New York: Kitchen Table: Women of Color Press, 1983), 264–74, quotation on 264.

5. Christine Jorgensen, *Christine Jorgensen: A Personal Autobiography* (New York: Paul S. Eriksson, 1967), 106.

6. Quoted in Elizabeth Siegel Watkins, *The Estrogen Elixir: A History of Hormone Replacement Therapy in America* (Baltimore: Johns Hopkins University Press, 2007), 187.

7. Susan Stryker, quoted in Deborah Rudacille, *The Riddle of Gender: Science, Activism, and Transgender Rights* (New York: Pantheon, 2006), 59.

8. Gianna E. Israel and Donald E. Tarver II, *Transgender Care: Recommended Guidelines, Practical Information, and Personal Accounts* (Philadelphia: Temple University Press, 2001).

9. Ian Hacking, "Kinds of People: Moving Targets," *Proceedings of the British Academy* 151 (2007): 285–318, quotation on 285.

10. Ibid., 285, 289, 293.

11. Ibid., 305.

12. Ibid., 296.

13. Peter D. Kramer, *Listening to Prozac: A Psychiatrist Explores Antidepressant Drugs and the Remaking of the Self* (New York: Viking, 1993), 19.

14. Katherine Sharpe, *Coming of Age on Zoloft: How Antidepressants Cheered Us Up, Let Us Down, and Changed Who We Are* (New York: Harper, 2012).

15. Kramer, *Listening to Prozac*, 10–19.

16. John Hoberman, *Testosterone Dreams: Rejuvenation, Aphrodisia, Doping* (Berkeley: University of California Press, 2005), 199.

17. Ibid., 180, 14.

18. Ibid., 19, 4.

19. I should note that Hacking's remarks on this matter were very brief, and his wording leaves open the possibility that I am taking his meaning in a direction he did not intend. Ian Hacking, *The Social Construction of What?* (Cambridge: Harvard University Press, 1999), 124.

20. Quoted in Christer Nordlund, "Endocrinology and Expectations in 1930s America: Louis Berman's Ideas on New Creations in Human Beings," *British Journal of History and Science* 40.1 (2007): 93.

21. Michel Foucault, *The History of Sexuality: An Introduction: Volume 1* (New York: Vintage, 1990), 101–2.

22. On the selling of depression as a disease see Ethan Watters, *Crazy Like Us: The Globalization of the American Psyche* (New York: Free Press, 2010), chap. 4.

23. Aditya Agrawal, "Illinois Bans Gay Conversion Therapy for Minors," *Time,* August 21, 2015.

Index

BOB OSTERTAG was born in Albuquerque in 1957. His work cannot easily be summarized or pigeon-holed. He has published twenty-four CDs of music, two DVDs, and five books. His writings on contemporary politics have been published on every continent and in many languages. He has performed at music, film, and multimedia festivals around the globe. His journalism covering the civil war in El Salvador in the 1980s continues to be cited by relevant scholarship today. His diverse music collaborators include the Kronos Quartet, avant-garder John Zorn, heavy metal star Mike Patton, jazz great Anthony Braxton, and transgender icon Justin Vivian Bond. He is rumored to have connections to the media guerrilla group The Yes Men. All of his recordings are free digital downloads under a Creative Commons license. Ostertag lives in San Francisco and is currently professor of cinema and digital media at the University of California at Davis.

CPSIA information can be obtained
at www.ICGtesting.com
Printed in the USA
BVOW00*1922231216
471764BV00003B/9/P